EMOTIONAL OVEREATING

Know the Triggers, Heal Your Mind, and Never Diet Again

MARCIA SIROTA, MD

The Praeger Series on Contemporary Health and Living
Julie K. Silver, MD, Series Editor

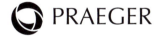 PRAEGER

AN IMPRINT OF ABC-CLIO, LLC
Santa Barbara, California • Denver, Colorado • Oxford, England

Copyright 2012 by Marcia Sirota, MD

All rights reserved. No part of this publication may be reproduced, stored in a retrieval system, or transmitted, in any form or by any means, electronic, mechanical, photocopying, recording, or otherwise, except for the inclusion of brief quotations in a review, without prior permission in writing from the publisher.

Library of Congress Cataloging-in-Publication Data

Sirota, Marcia.
  Emotional overeating : know the triggers, heal your mind, and never diet again /
Marcia Sirota.
      p. cm. — (The Praeger series on contemporary health and living)
    Includes index.
    ISBN 978-1-4408-0401-4 (hardback) — ISBN 978-1-4408-0402-1 (ebook)
1. Compulsive eating.   2. Eating disorders.   3. Food habits—Psychological aspects.   I. Title.
    RC552.C65S49   2012
    616.85′26—dc23   2012014066

ISBN: 978-1-4408-0401-4

EISBN: 978-1-4408-0402-1

16   15   14   13   12   1   2   3   4   5

This book is also available on the World Wide Web as an eBook.

Visit www.abc-clio.com for details.
Praeger

An Imprint of ABC-CLIO, LLC

ABC-CLIO, LLC
130 Cremona Drive, P.O. Box 1911
Santa Barbara, California 93116-1911

This book is printed on acid-free paper ∞

Manufactured in the United States of America

CONTENTS

Series Foreword

Contemporary Health and Living

Over the past 100 years, there have been incredible medical breakthroughs that have prevented or cured illness in billions of people and helped many more improve their health while living with chronic conditions. A few of the most important 20th century discoveries include antibiotics, organ transplants, and vaccines. The 21st century has already heralded important new treatments including such things as a vaccine to prevent human papillomavirus from infecting and potentially leading to cervical cancer in women. Polio is on the verge of being eradicated worldwide, making it only the second infectious disease behind smallpox to ever be erased as a human health threat.

In this series, experts from many disciplines share with readers important information about medical issues—including problems, symptoms, diseases and whenever possible, solutions. Disseminating this information will help individuals to recognize things that impact their health and that of loved ones. Researchers may use these books to determine where there are gaps in our current knowledge, and policy makers may be able to better assess the most pressing needs in healthcare. The overarching goal of this series of books is to inform people about important issues in modern medicine.

Series Editor Julie K. Silver, MD
Assistant Professor
Harvard Medical School
Department of Physical Medicine and Rehabilitation

Preface: A True Story about the Disappearance of 100 Pounds

This is a story about two of my first psychotherapy patients. I was new to this type of work, having begun my practice as a family doctor. Due to my lack of experience, I didn't yet have a sense of how the therapy I was offering would affect the people I was seeing, or what outcomes I could expect.

Over time, I saw that many of my patients had symptoms of post-traumatic stress disorder, and that I had a knack for helping these people. They were mostly women who'd been abused or somehow traumatized as children.

Kate and Jenny were two such women. They came to see me in 1991: Kate in the winter, and Jenny in the spring. These women had a number of problems in common, including relationship and self-esteem issues and long-term struggles with their weight. They'd both tried dieting many times, and neither had succeeded in keeping off any weight that they'd lost.

In most other ways, these women were very different from each other: Kate was in her mid-30s, petite, blonde, upper-middle class, and very proper and reserved. She was single and worked in a conservative office environment. Jenny, on the other hand, was a tall, fiftyish, auburn-haired free spirit who dressed flamboyantly. She was married for many years and had one grown child.

Kate had a tragic history. She'd been molested by a close friend of the family who'd been her babysitter when she was young. She'd never been able to tell anyone about what had happened because in her family, things like that simply weren't discussed.

Jenny had a somewhat less horrific past. Her self-absorbed, neglectful hippy parents didn't notice that her stepfather's oldest son had begun smoking marijuana with her when she turned 11, eventually introducing her to cocaine, and to sex. The sex and the drug use went on for years, until Jenny ended up in a rehab center for a year and a half in her early 20s. She was able to stop using drugs by the time she turned 30, married, and had begun to make a life for herself.

Both these women had a lot of pain and shame deep down. Both overate on a regular basis, and had pretty much given up on losing weight. I made a decision at the start of therapy with both of them not to talk about their eating or weight. It was such a fraught topic that it didn't seem like it would be helpful to go there.

My sense was that neither one needed to feel like she was being pushed in her therapy to focus on something about which she felt so helpless and hopeless. Both of them were so wounded and emotionally fragile that I felt we had enough to work on just dealing with their current life problems and past traumas. Besides, I wasn't entirely confident that we could do much about the eating or their weight since both women had been struggling unsuccessfully with these problems for years. They didn't bring up the issue, so I left it alone.

Another reason for my choosing to put aside the issues of eating and weight in my therapy with Kate and Jenny was because of a pattern I'd noticed among my patients: many of them had insight into their emotional problems, but this insight hadn't helped them make any meaningful changes in their lives. Both Kate and Jenny understood that they ate for emotional reasons, but this understanding hadn't enabled either to change her behavior. I felt it would only create frustration if I focused on them developing more insight, when it wasn't yet clear idea how I might put this insight to good use.

Here were two women, each of whom understood that she was engaging in "emotional eating" and knew all there was to know about nutrition and health, but was significantly overweight. It was a crucial issue in each of their lives, but it was an area so charged with shame and hopelessness that neither could bring herself to discuss it in therapy. I chose to concentrate on helping them face their past traumas so they could begin the process of healing.

Surprisingly, after I'd been working with each woman individually for a number of months, I started to notice that both Kate and Jenny were beginning to lose weight. Neither of them had been dieting, but within a few weeks, first Jenny and then Kate walked into my office, sat down, and announced that she had, for the first time in a long time, lost some weight.

It was a small amount in both cases, and I didn't want to put too much attention on it. I didn't want to interfere with the unconscious process that must be happening, so I simply acknowledged the change. As the weeks went by and they came in for their sessions, I could see that each woman was growing thinner and thinner. It became apparent that the weight was not just coming off but staying off in both cases, so after several months I finally asked them how much they'd lost. Each woman triumphantly answered, "fifty pounds!"

Was this a weird coincidence? How was it that these two women could each lose so much weight, without trying? They had in common their painful childhoods and current therapy, but was there something specific about Kate and Jenny that I wasn't aware of? It began to dawn on me that without ever directly dealing with their eating or weight issues in therapy, these women had succeeded in doing the one thing that had eluded them all of their adult lives.

Even more significantly, these two women had also lost the urge to over-eat. In fact, both of them had at about the same time stopped their constant obsessing about overeating and weight, as well as their compulsive seesawing of overeating then food restricting, and the pounds had just fallen away. After years of agonizing over this problem and struggling in vain to lose 15 or 20 pounds, both women had shed 50 pounds in a relatively short period of time without effort.

As time passed and the pounds fell away, I noticed that both Kate and Jenny would walk into my office with smiles on their faces. Both were bemused about their seemingly magical weight loss, and although initially it wasn't clear what was happening, we were all delighted.

I was very interested in what they were experiencing because it went against my psychotherapy training. I was taught that you deal with an issue to make it better, and here, the one issue we hadn't dealt with was the one at which both women had excelled.

I thought a lot about Kate and Jenny. Before this, I'd only seen women become thinner after fighting hard for every 2-pound drop, constantly scrutinizing their eating habits and their scales, but here, 100 pounds had just disappeared!

Eventually, I realized that one reason why Kate and Jenny had lost the weight was precisely because we *hadn't* talked about it in our therapy sessions. When we did begin to look at the subject of food and weight, it became clear that these things weren't the real problem, but a symptom of deeper wounds that needed to be healed.

By not insisting that the women deal with their overeating, each woman was able to just do her therapy. The work we did together on their underlying emotional issues enabled both women to lose weight, keep it off, and normalize their relationship with their body and food. Without our trying to do so, these women were cured.

ACKNOWLEDGMENTS

A book about compulsive eating and the women who engage in it isn't something that arises out of thin air. First and foremost, I have to thank all the women who've attended my workshops and general practice and who've inspired me to put into writing what I've learned from them. I'd also like to thank all those who assisted in bringing this book to completion. Thank you to my readers, including Ann Rauhala, Dr. Teri Richard, and Jon Oelrich and most especially Jay Tropianskaya, who read the enormous first draft and still found good things to say about it. Thanks to Beverly Slopen and Nick Garrison for helpful technical advice. I am very grateful to my teachers, most especially Drs. William Fried and Marvin Lipkowitz at Maimonides Medical Center in Brooklyn, New York, who provided me with a first-rate education. I'll never forget Dr. Lipkowitz for reminding me that it was my love for my patients that would do them the most good. Thanks to Myra and Mel Tennenbaum for their unconditional love and support. Many thanks to the Wolffs for keeping me well fueled for the journey, and to my editor, Debbie Carvalko, whose generous help and guidance made this book a reality. Finally, gracias to RNP, for inspiring me to write. *La limonata esta rica.*

1

COMPULSIVE EATING: THE BIG PICTURE

It seems as though we've become a society of addicts. Everywhere we turn, we're confronted with evidence of our rampant addictions. TV shows like *Celebrity Rehab* and *Intervention* have become commonplace, gambling is available online and at the corner grocery store, pornography is the number-one item downloaded on computers, and surgical centers specializing in lap band and bariatric procedures are more and more commonplace.

In particular, we've become a nation of compulsive overeaters, hyper-focused on everything having to do with food and eating. An epidemic of obesity is upon us, with wide-reaching implications to our health, economy, and culture, but how did we get here? Is this a new phenomenon or part of a cycle of behavior that reflects our basic human nature?

According to the most recent statistics from the Centers for Disease Control and Prevention, just over one-third of the adults in the United States are obese. In Canada, the rate is closer to one-fourth but it's increasing steadily. Currently, in the United States, there isn't one state in which less than 15 percent of the population is obese.

Obesity-related medical costs in the United States in 2008 topped $140 million and third-party payers spent more than $1,400 dollars more for obese individuals than they did for normal-weight people that same year. The rate of type 2 diabetes (an illness directly correlated with being overweight) has significantly increased in prevalence over the past 18 years. According to the World Health Organization, there are more than 1 billion overweight adults on the planet today, of which at least 300 million are obese.

It's clear that the rates of obesity and obesity-related illness are skyrocketing, but how do we make sense of these data? We need to look at the many factors that have come together to create our current epidemic.

I think that the North American obesity problem today is a result of the combination of three main factors: (1) greater access to inexpensive food that is densely packed with poor-quality calories; (2) a more sedentary lifestyle where people drive instead of walking and spend hours in front of the TV set or the computer screen; and (3) a pervasive state of unhappiness arising from an excess of neglect, abuse, and trauma in childhood as well as a general lack of meaning, purpose, and interpersonal connectedness in adult life.

Eating is a complex behavior. It's driven not only by hunger but also by the interplay of numerous biological, psychological, emotional, nutritional, social, and economic factors. The craving for a cookie, for example, doesn't just come from the urge to eat something sweet but is meaningful, in that it reflects not just the person's desire for the treat but also their yearning for love, comfort, belonging, emotional numbing, even social status.

Food has always been of the utmost importance, but today it's become so overvalued that we can't stop thinking about it, let alone consuming it. We've become obsessed with food, eating, and our body shape and size. We're compulsive in our eating behavior, whether this means binge eating, restricting, or purging, or a combination of these. Our behavior with regard to food is contradictory, often with the same person bouncing between compulsive overeating and compulsive dieting, all the while maintaining an obsessive preoccupation with what's being consumed.

Many people today are writing about the problems that result from a sedentary lifestyle and calorie-rich, poor-quality food. I'll leave it up to them to explain why high-fructose corn syrup and hours spent in front of a computer screen are conducive to an expanding waistline. What I want to focus on is the way our childhood difficulties and adult unhappiness come together to create the perfect circumstances in which compulsive eating and obesity are the only logical response.

Addiction has become so prevalent today and is such a difficult-to-treat problem that theorists have proclaimed it to be a disease, akin to cancer or hypothyroidism. I have always found this idea to be facile and unhelpful. Some researchers even talk about an "addictive personality" whereby the individual is intelligent, creative, charismatic, and visionary; seeks thrills and novelty; is driven to succeed; is innovative; challenges the status quo; and takes risks.[1]

While it's true that some individuals are more prone to addiction due to a case of "faulty wiring" in their brain where they more actively seek out pleasurable sensations due to an inadequate response to pleasurable activities, this alone doesn't account for why so many of us engage in so many different addictions. In fact, according to David J. Linden, a Johns Hopkins-based professor of neuroscience, genetic factors only account for 40–60 percent of the risk of addiction.[2]

Rather than seeing addiction as a disease, and overeating and obesity as problems that are beyond the control of the affected individual, I look at overeating, obesity, and addiction in general as a way of dealing with two fundamental aspects of unhappiness: childhood hurts, losses, and unmet needs and adult suffering, whether conscious or unconscious.

I think that we engage in addictions as a way to compensate both for the hurts and losses of our early years and for what's missing in our adult lives today. As I'll discuss in detail further on in the book, these two problems are at the root of addiction and are the key to the treatment of every addiction, including overeating and obesity.

If it were up to me I'd recommend that we throw out all our old ideas of how to treat not just overeating and obesity but all addictions, because it's clear that the current approaches aren't effective. In my work with women who overeat, the focus has never been on the weight or the diet but on the real underlying reasons why a person is driven to eat compulsively and to carry extra weight.

In the following chapter, I'll talk about what I think true happiness is, how we lost track of it, and how we can find it again. I'll discuss how we engage in overeating as a way to compensate for our inner sense of emptiness and alienation and how we can heal this condition without resorting to food.

FREEDOM THROUGH EMOTIONAL HEALING

If you're an overeater, you know that being heavy and *eating excessively* aren't your only problems. In fact, you can't stop *thinking* about food and weight. What you want to eat, what you think you should eat, what you just ate, what you shouldn't have eaten, and each pound up and down on the scale are all dwelt on in minute detail. Obsessing about food, weight, and dieting is a major part of the problem as opposed to any part of the solution. One of the main problems with dieting is that it encourages this obsessing. A real solution should enable you to normalize your relationship with food and your body and turn your attention to the things that will bring you true happiness and fulfillment.

Both compulsive eating and compulsive food restricting (dieting) cause a behavioral vicious circle, in which overeating leads to remorse, self-recrimination, heightened obsessions, and then to further overeating. Not only does this vicious circle fail to address the problem, but it also creates enormous emotional suffering. You may or may not be dealing with the health or social consequences of overeating but if you're currently dieting, you're probably suffering from a constant preoccupation with food and weight.

It's possible to spend all your free time focused on the ins and outs of your diet and weight issues. People think that they don't have an eating disorder if their weight is normal for their age and body type, but it's not your size that's indicative of the problem; it's the degree to which you think obsessively and behave compulsively with regard to food and your weight. No matter what your size is, if you can't stop thinking about eating and weight and can't stop compulsively indulging or restricting, then you're unhappily locked in the prison of food addiction. Until you've let go of the obsessive thinking and compulsive behaviors associated with disordered eating, you'll never be happy or free.

Dina's Story

Dina, a 30-year-old patient of mine who struggles with compulsive eating, shared a story recently about a friend, Mimi, who's very thin but extremely pre-occupied with what she eats. Mimi's anxiety is so extreme that she becomes visibly distressed if she's encouraged to eat something she thinks she "shouldn't" eat. Mimi is the same age as Dina, and could maintain a healthy weight by eating normal amounts of regular food. Instead, she consumes a severely re-stricted range of low-calorie foods doled out in tiny portions.

Dina also obsesses about how much she weighs and what she should and shouldn't eat. As opposed to the overly controlled Mimi, Dina's eating and weight are out of control. In therapy, Dina realized that she and Mimi are mir-ror images of one another and that Mimi's situation is not an improvement on hers. There's no success in being thin and miserably preoccupied. Both women have an eating disorder that makes them terribly unhappy. Whether heavy or skinny, overindulging or restricting, the worlds of both women are very small because neither can think of anything else besides food and weight.

Real freedom from the prison of disordered eating is being able to let go of the preoccupation with food and body; it's having the time, energy, and mental clarity to pursue the activities and relationships that will bring true happiness and fulfillment. These things ought to be the real goals of healing, as opposed to achieving any particular weight.

Dina, at more than 250 pounds, will be better off than Mimi at 100 pounds if she can let go of her obsessive thinking and compulsive behavior with re-gard to eating and weight. The obsessing keeps all of this a charged subject and in the forefront of consciousness, where it increases the urge to overeat. If Dina were to put her attention on the real solutions to her problem, she'd be able to stop obsessing about eating and her body, her relationship with food and weight would normalize, and she'd no longer be compelled to indulge or restrict with regard to food. Releasing the obsession means freedom from the compulsion, and if she were able to do so, Dina's weight would come off without effort.

The problem with diets is that they keep you focused on the false solution of food restriction. You're so preoccupied with food and weight that you're unable to consider what's really driving you to overeat and how to effectively deal with your cravings. Diets would have you avoiding certain foods instead of indulging in them, but you're still caught up in compulsive patterns of be-havior. Diets also draw your energy from the things in your life that could be meaningful and could contribute to your healing. Letting go of dieting helps you begin to search for the real cause of your overeating and for meaningful sources of healing. Only this will allow you to lose weight and free yourself of your obsessions and compulsive behaviors forever.

So, how do you know that you have disordered eating? First and foremost, you need to look at how and why you eat. You might be someone who just eats a little bit more than you should. Maybe you regularly indulge in an after-dinner treat. Maybe you overdo it at a restaurant, a party, or a buffet. You might not be that much overweight—maybe just 5 or 10 pounds more than you'd like, but because of your tendency to overeat just that little bit, the extra pounds don't go away. Maybe even you've been gaining a few pounds each year.

Alternatively, you could be someone who eats slightly too-large portions on a regular basis. Perhaps your stomach has stretched and it takes more for you to feel full. Maybe, as a result, you feel hungry much of the time. You may engage in evening binges, eating a large amount of food in a short period of time, not even tasting what you've swallowed, only to repeat this behavior the next day.

Whichever scenario describes you best, if you're even a little bit out of control of your eating, then you're someone for whom food isn't solely a source of enjoyable nutrition but is to some degree a charged subject. If you have trouble controlling what you put in your mouth and, especially, if you're preoccupied with the whole topic of food, weight, eating, and dieting, you have an issue with eating. Those who overindulge a little bit and are just a bit overweight and those who overeat a lot and are significantly overweight aren't that different.

What differentiates a mild or moderate overeater from a more serious one is related to two fundamental factors: the degree to which you've been wounded emotionally and the degree to which food has become the solution to your emotional needs. Essentially, the presence of any amount of neglect, abuse, loss, or trauma in your childhood has left you with the emotional wounds of *unhealed pain and unmet needs,* which persist in adult life; it's these wounds that drive you to overeat in search of compensation and healing.

You might have had reasonably good parents who loved you the best they could and who had the best intentions for you. In that case, you'll have been spared the worst type of wounding (from severe abuse or neglect) and your milder eating and weight issues will be proportional to your milder unresolved emotional issues.

It's not unheard of, however, that people with loving, supportive families could develop wounds from childhood traumas related to being mistreated or even abused by a teacher or a coach, for example, or by being bullied or tormented by peers. You could have experienced the loss of a family member, a serious illness in the family, the suicide of a close relative, or the substance abuse of a parent.

It's also possible that you grew up in a situation that was emotionally wounding because of traumatic political, social, or environmental events. You don't have to look to your parents alone to explain why you might have a problem with eating or weight.

If you grew up with loving, caring parents, but experienced some traumatic childhood events, you might have internalized enough self-confidence and self-love that you made it to adulthood with only minor problems, as manifested by a mild overeating/weight problem. If your parents weren't as loving or supportive, then whether or not you experienced other upsetting events in childhood, you'll be more likely to have developed an eating problem.

Dr. Vincent J. Felitti of the Department of Preventative Medicine at the Kaiser Permanente Medical Care Program in San Diego California describes how he and his colleagues did a population-based analysis of over 17,000 healthy, middle-class American adults to explore the relationship of what he calls "adverse childhood experiences" to the development of addictions.[3] His conclusion was that childhood experiences of hurt, loss, trauma, or neglect contribute to the development of addiction, whereby a greater variety of adverse experiences is correlated with a greater likelihood of having one or more addictions. Through this study, Dr. Felitti recognized that addictions are unconscious coping devices as opposed to a brain disease, a chemical imbalance, or a case of faulty genetics.[4]

When I read this paper and many of the other writings derived from the Adverse Childhood Experiences study, I was gratified to see that this well-founded research corroborated my many years of clinical observations. I came to my conclusions based on case after case of patients who suffered from one, two, or more addictions, who had a history of these adverse childhood experiences, and who were cured of their addictions by dealing with their unhealed emotional wounds and unmet emotional needs. As Dr. Felitti points out, these types of experiences are a lot more common than we'd like to think, but both the affected individuals as well as the clinicians treating them have a strong resistance to recognizing this truth.[5] If you're to overcome your own compulsive eating or other addiction(s), you'll have to open your mind to the possibility that you've suffered at least one of these adverse events (more if your addictions are severe or multiple) when you were growing up.

Another factor that plays a role in the degree to which you're not in control of your eating behavior is the way that food was used in your family and community. If there was a lot of emphasis on food and eating and especially if food was used as a substitute for love, then you'll have an overvalued idea of food. If food was too important to your parents, and if they modeled to you through their behavior that eating was difficult to do in moderation, you'll have internalized this message and will find yourself struggling to control your own eating as an adult. If one or both parents shamed you over what you ate or tried to control your eating, telling you all the time what you "should" or "shouldn't" be eating, food would have become a highly charged substance that you'd find impossible to resist as an adult.

Food is the first thing that soothed and comforted you and the first thing that your parents gave you as an expression of their love and care. This makes it a powerful symbolic entity. It represents love and healing in every culture, and is the first and most common substance that a person turns to when she's looking for soothing and nurturing. Some type of food is going to be available in most places around the world, at least some of the time. Here in the West, an abundant supply of food is available at all times. Furthermore, eating is legal, relatively safe, and can be done in the privacy of your own home. It's easy to see why a person would turn to overeating to deal with emotional needs.

On the other hand, if your community or family didn't place any special emphasis on food, it might not be the main way in which you look for nurturing or healing. Maybe one parent was a drinker or a compulsive shopper. Maybe in your community, gambling was highly regarded as an escape from stress or perhaps you witnessed people turning to drugs to ease their pain. If food was not a charged subject and the emphasis instead was on one or more of these other things, then you could have easily learned to use something other than food to deal with your unresolved emotional needs.

It's not uncommon that someone with a mild overeating problem has a more significant issue with spending, drinking, or smoking, for example. Alternatively, you could have several mild addictions that combine to make a more serious problem. Whether overeating is your only problem or one of several issues, and whether overeating is a minor or more significant issue for you, you're going to have to face the fact that your addictions have arisen from emotional wounds that need to be addressed.

Think of it this way: dealing with your eating problem could be a way for you to finally become conscious about unresolved childhood issues. By facing and dealing with your habit of overeating, you'll be able to achieve real emotional healing. Once this is accomplished, you'll be able to access the energy that was being channeled into attempts at controlling your eating and weight, and redirect it into more meaningful and fulfilling activities. Also, the same emotional healing that allows you to let go of your minor eating problem will free you from any other addiction you might have. Understanding the meaning of your disordered eating can turn into an opportunity to deal, finally, with these other issues.

Over the years, during my work with women who overeat, I've noticed a shocking trend: *the after-diet weight gain.* The truth is that many of my patients gained more weight after dieting than they had originally lost and ended up heavier than when they began. After many tries at dieting, some of these women—who'd started off only mildly overweight—actually *dieted themselves fat.*

ELOISE'S STORY

Eloise, a vivacious 50-something professional woman, first took up dieting at the age of 17 when she was 5'5" and weighed 135 pounds. Her mother had been pressuring her to lose weight, telling Eloise that she was "too big." Since that first diet 35 years ago, Eloise has tried the low-carb diet, the soup diet, the grapefruit diet, and many others without success. At the beginning of her therapy with me, she weighed over 200 pounds and was suffering from high blood pressure, diabetes, and elevated cholesterol. Because of these health problems, her family doctor had her taking multiple medications. The same doctor had sent her to me as a last resort, as Eloise by now had completely given up on ever losing weight. The hope was that by working with me, Eloise might be able to lose the few pounds that would make a big difference to her health. Eloise told me that every time she went on a diet, she'd begin to lose some weight but then the weight would all come back, and then some. Essentially, Eloise had dieted her way to her current health crisis.

There are a number of problems with the whole notion of dieting. Here are a few reasons why I think diets can't really help a woman take weight off and keep it off permanently.

1. Dieting is a symptomatic treatment that never takes into consideration the root causes of compulsive eating.
2. Dieting imposes painful restrictions on someone who already feels deprived and unfulfilled.
3. Dieting depends on the exercise of extreme willpower in someone who has already demonstrated difficulties with self-control.
4. Dieting deprives the person of the (albeit false) solution to their unmet needs and unhealed wounds without providing a viable alternative.
5. Dieting doesn't address the fact that overeating is a powerfully self-reinforcing behavior.
6. Dieting has been shown to lead to weight gain.
7. Dieting doesn't take into account the powerful psychological forces that drive compulsive eating behaviors.

Now that I've outlined these problems, let me go into more detail about them.

Dieting doesn't deal with the reasons why you overeat, and until you understand why you're driven to eat compulsively, you'll be hard-pressed to find a solution. Dieting deals with the symptoms of the problem—overeating and being overweight—but not with the emotional issues that drive you to eat excessively or to carry extra weight. Forcing yourself to eat less will be a losing battle, because these issues won't go away just because you're dieting. In fact, dieting makes things worse.

Unless you understand what the food does for you and what the weight *means* to you and how you can replace overeating and being overweight with something better and healthier, it will be impossible to let go of the problem. If there's an unconscious reason why you're holding on to the extra weight and you begin to diet without addressing the psychological aspects of what you're giving up, any weight that you've lost will cause you so much stress or anxiety that you'll need to put it back on.

LUCINDA'S STORY

A few years ago, I worked with a researcher in her 30s named Lucinda. She was a lovely and extremely overweight young woman who once shared with me how in her 20s she'd gone to an expensive diet clinic and had lost

100 pounds. Lucinda had believed that she wanted to be thinner and had spent a lot of money at this clinic in order to do so. Surprisingly, she became so anxious in her new, smaller body that she couldn't put the weight back on quickly enough. Lucinda hadn't considered that the extra weight had a psychological function for her. In fact, deep down, Lucinda didn't really want to lose the weight, because for reasons that were still unclear to her, she needed to be heavy. Until she understood why she had to hold onto the weight, she was never going to keep off any that she might lose.

Dieting by definition involves restricting or limiting certain types of foods, portion size, or daily amounts of food. Overeaters are unconsciously using extra food to deal with unresolved emotional hurts, losses, and needs. Any diet you try will cause feelings of emotional deprivation, frustration, emptiness, and stress, which you'll eventually compensate for through further overeating.

The act of dieting requires an enormous amount of willpower and self-control. Overeating becomes a habitual way of coping with unconscious issues. You can try to force yourself to change this habit, but there's a strong unconscious reason for you to have started. Willpower alone won't be enough for you to succeed. In fact, depending too much on willpower almost always leads to what I call "willpower burnout," where your self-control dissolves. It takes too much effort to keep forcing yourself to lose weight and keep it off. When you become exhausted and your willpower runs out, you'll inevitably go back to coping through overeating.

You might ask, "is there any role for willpower?" and the answer is, "yes," but it has to be combined with conscious awareness of your reasons for over-eating. For example, if you tend to overeat at parties and you realize that it's because you get anxious in social situations, you can use this awareness to remind yourself that you're going to the party to enjoy yourself. If it's not fun, you can give yourself permission to leave. Armed with this self-knowledge and self-trust, you can use your willpower to keep focused on your needs and feelings at the party. If you're not having fun, there's an alternative to spending your entire time at the buffet table.

Dieting takes away something that's essential without replacing it. It makes you give up the food you're convinced you need and replaces it with a smaller quantity of less palatable food. It makes you give up overeating when you feel stressed, empty, lonely, irritable, or bored without giving you a better way of coping. It takes away a comforting habit that, deep down, you're convinced you can't live without. In fact, dieting can make you feel so deprived that it could lead to other problems.

JOSIE'S STORY

One of my patients, an accountant named Josie, confessed that she'd developed a shopping addiction while she was dieting. She began buying herself things as a way of dealing with the experience of frustration and powerlessness brought on by dieting. She spent a lot of money but her diet still failed because shopping didn't compensate for what the diet took away. In the end, Josie weighed the same as she did at the beginning of her diet, but also faced an additional debt problem. Meanwhile, neither dieting nor shopping was meeting her real needs.

When it comes to your behavior, you have two minds: the *conscious awareness* you believe is responsible for your behavior and the *unconscious needs, feelings, and urges,* which are responsible for a far greater number of choices than you might imagine. In fact, human beings are often driven by unconscious processes, and certain behaviors, like addictions, are always driven by your unconscious mind. It's an instinctual survival mechanism to automatically bury memories, feelings, or needs in the unconscious if they're frightening, confusing, or painful. They stay buried until you become aware of them and are comfortable enough to address them.

Humans can have very limited conscious awareness, with many of our actions arising from buried needs and urges. Fortunately, it's possible to become a lot more aware of what's going on under the surface, and to make conscious choices of how to act based on what you know about your feelings and needs. It is possible for you to move memories and feelings out of your unconscious and into your conscious awareness, much like moving files on a computer. Becoming more conscious requires a certain amount of work. I'll describe the process in more detail later on.

As I mentioned previously, I see addiction not as a disease but as a repetitive behavior driven by the unconscious need to deal with unmet emotional needs or unhealed emotional wounds that exist because of difficult childhood experiences. Addiction is a repetitive act for two reasons: one, because you're desperately craving relief or fulfillment and are convinced that addiction is the solution, and two, the addictive behavior appears to satisfy your needs but in reality isn't actually capable of giving you what you seek, so you keep engaging in it, hoping that maybe next time it'll work.

Compulsive eating comes from an unconscious need for emotional healing and nurturing. Because of things you experienced while growing up, and because of the messages you've received about food and eating, you've come to feel deep down, that eating is the way to nurture or heal yourself. If you're unaware of what's going on in your unconscious mind and don't know of a better way to deal with these issues, you won't be able to make the choice to give up overeating and go for what you really need.

If you're unconscious about what's driving your addiction and don't understand that there's something better out there that can replace overeating; something that actually meets your emotional needs, dieting will leave a big empty space inside you that must be filled. Like I said, this is why so many people who've been dieting will go back to overeating or find different ways to deal with this empty feeling.

Many people begin to drink or smoke heavily or turn to gambling, compulsive shopping, or using illegal or prescription drugs to make up for what's missing once they've given up overeating. In this way, most addictions or compulsive behaviors are interchangeable, because they serve the same purpose: to deal with unmet emotional needs and unhealed emotional wounds. Just like what happened with Josie, none of these activities satisfy, so you could conceivably go from one addiction to the other or accumulate several new addictions until you finally address your real needs and feelings.

Overeating is a self-perpetuating activity. Every time you overeat you get just enough soothing or distraction from painful feelings that you'll experience it as somewhat positive. Your brain has pleasure centers that respond to positive experiences by releasing chemicals that make you want to continue these experiences. The brain also has centers that register a feeling of happy satisfaction when you're physically full. Under normal circumstances, these two centers work together, so that you're driven to eat because it's pleasurable, but then feel the urge to stop when you're full. Overeating is a positive enough experience for you to want to continue, but not so positive as to make you satisfied enough to stop. That's because of two things: regular overeating overstimulates your pleasure centers, eventually making them increasingly less sensitive to the pleasurable feelings associated with eating. Ironically, the more you eat, the less you enjoy it and the more short lived the pleasure. You need to eat more and more for it to feel as pleasurable as it once did. Like with drugs or alcohol, this is the physiological experience of tolerance.

The second reason is that you'll eventually short-circuit your brain center that registers the sensation of fullness (the satiety center) if you continue to eat after it has indicated that you're full. No matter how much you've eaten, you'll continue to feel hungry. You'll stop eating only when you're uncomfortable. So, overeating leaves you not only too full but also frustrated. You've eaten as much as you can take in but don't feel happy or fulfilled. Sadly, because of increased tolerance for the pleasure-sensation of overeating and the dulling of the satiety center, overeating leads to more overeating.

Dieting can make you fat. If you suddenly begin to restrict calories, your metabolism will respond by slowing down as a biological survival mechanism to prevent starvation. At the end of the diet, when you try to go back to "normal" eating, your metabolism won't speed up because it's still reacting to the previous lack of calories and to the possibility that soon you might begin to starve again. Even after you've started eating your "maintenance" diet, your basal metabolic rate remains "down-shifted" in response to the lengthy period of caloric restriction, so the same amount of calories that would cause a non-dieter to maintain her weight will cause you to gain weight. This drives you to go back on the diet, which further slows your metabolic rate so that the more you diet the less you're able to eat without gaining weight.

Even if you begin to exercise to increase your basal metabolic rate, it will take some time for things to go back to normal. Initially, you'll have to work much harder than a non-dieter and eat much less, just to keep from gaining weight. Ironically, the more you exercise, the more you'll increase your appetite. You'll have to exercise constantly while constantly being hungry, just to maintain your original, heavier weight. The more you exercise, though, the hungrier you'll get. Eventually, many people can't resist overeating to satisfy this intense, exercise-induced hunger.

Furthermore, if you're exercising heavily but aren't taking in proper nutrition in the form of complex carbohydrates, good fats, and protein, your body will become stressed. Levels of the stress hormone cortisol become elevated when people exercise without ingesting sufficient good-quality calories. This causes the breakdown of muscle tissue. Increased levels of cortisol are also responsible for increasing body fat. Regular, moderate exercise gradually increases the basal metabolic rate, has minimal effects on the appetite, and is excellent for your health. Exercising excessively while restricting food intake will give you the opposite results to what you were hoping for.

Dieting always involves an unconscious inner conflict between three different parts of your psyche. Sigmund Freud calls these three aspects of the psyche the *Id, Ego,* and *Superego.* Today, they can be known as the *child within,* the *adult self,* and the *internalized parent.* The child part of the psyche is the persistent presence of the child you once were. It carries the emotional wounds of the past and wants to overeat for healing and compensation. The adult self is the you of today that wants to be free of the problem but may not yet be strong enough to do this, and the internalized parent is the accumulation of all the parental and societal voices you've taken in over the years that tells you that you're fat and you must diet. Further on I'll explain how these three parts of the psyche interact and their roles in compulsive overeating.

I have a patient named Joanne who eats celery compulsively. She can go through 15 stalks in an evening. Another patient, Eleanor, habitually eats two pints of vanilla ice cream on a Sunday afternoon, and Josie can go through a dozen donuts when she gets home from work. At least once a week, Jocelyn, another patient of mine, eats an entire extra-large pizza. Obviously, none of these women are eating like this out of physical hunger. In fact, after they're done, the thing all these women have in common is a sense of remorse for having overeaten. This behavior has nothing to do with appetite and everything to do with emotional needs.

So how do you go from this behavior to eating with consciousness? The answer may not be easy, but it's quite simple: eat as your adult self and not as the child within. I'll explain what I mean: the child within sees eating as the solution to her problem of being wounded emotionally. She experiences an overpowering physical hunger, but it's really an emotional one. The child within seeks healing and fulfillment, seeing food as the cure for what ails her.

In the inner conflict, the child within is the impulsive, illogical, primitive part of the psyche. It's convinced that food equals love, comfort, or healing. This part drives you to overeat, in the hope that eventually, the child within will find what she needs in food. The internalized parent is the negative, demanding part of your psyche that tells you what you "should" and "shouldn't" do; it criticizes and shames you for being overweight and blames you for "being out of control."

The adult self should be what you identify with today, but when there have been significant childhood wounds, the child part of the psyche remains in the forefront of consciousness as its agenda to find healing and nurturing takes precedence. Unlike the illogical child self, the adult part of the psyche has the ability to make rational choices about how you eat, but only if this is your main identity and you don't allow the impulsive child within or the controlling internalized parent to be in charge of your eating.

The child within is driven to overeat by an overwhelming need to deal with emotional wounds. The internalized parent insists on dieting, and the child within, fearing further deprivation, resists. The power struggle between these two parts of the psyche is so intense that there's little room for any input from the rational adult self. The internalized parent is pushing the child within to restrict food, and the child is pushing back. Because these two parts of your psyche have locked horns, the adult self can't be in charge of your eating be-havior and you remain at an impasse, losing and then regaining any weight you might have lost.

The inner conflict is more likely if you've grown up with parents or guard-ians who, because of their abuse or neglect, didn't enable you to develop a strong, consistent adult identity that could take charge of the child and par-ent parts of your psyche. A strong adult self would take responsibility for the nurturing of the child within and healing of its wounds and would reject the negative parental messages.

The act of dieting pits the child and parental parts of your psyche against each other. The child might initially try to please the parent, allowing you to comply for a time with the diet plan, but this usually won't last because there's no pleasing the ultracritical internalized parent, and because the child within eventually tires of trying to do so.

The adult self wants to be healthy and free of addiction. If you begin to identify as an adult, dieting won't be necessary because you'll take responsibil-ity for resolving the problem of your unmet needs and unhealed wounds of childhood, as opposed to just dealing with the symptoms. Being a strong adult means discovering the unconscious needs and feelings that are driving your overeating behavior and making conscious, responsible choices about healing your wounds and giving the child within what she really needs. Dieting has absolutely nothing to do with this.

For all the reasons I've mentioned, diets can't possibly work. But still, women (and men) are regularly being enticed by the false promises of the diet industry. In order to get women to spend their money, it tells them, "it's your fault that you've chosen the wrong diet," or "you're a failure because you lack self-discipline." The truth is you can try diet after diet, blaming each one for its failure. You can get angry at yourself for being "weak," "self-indulgent," or "out of control." You could even despair over your inability to lose weight and keep it off. The truth is that the problem isn't with you or even the particular diet, but with the entire concept of dieting.

The diet industry makes billions of dollars every year, mainly from women's overeating problems. It's been capitalizing on your desperation for many years, selling you expensive and useless diets but it has never once taken responsibility and admitted that dieting failures represent a flaw in the whole concept of dieting. You can choose, right now, to stop allowing the diet industry to exploit your desperation to lose weight. If even one of these diets were successful, it would have cornered the market and the others would have ceased to exist. The fact that there are so many programs available and that women often try several of them means that none actually work.

A review of 31 studies on diet outcomes done by Traci Mann, Janet Tomiyama, and their colleagues at the University of California, Los Angeles, found that despite the fact that most diets lead to short-term weight loss, these losses not only weren't maintained but the weight was regained in the great majority of cases, often resulting in the dieter weighing more than they did before beginning the diet.[6] Their conclusion was that the dieters would have been better off not to have gone on a diet at all,[7] as their bodies wouldn't have incurred the stress of repeated weight loss and gains.

The clinical evidence as well as the research amply demonstrates that diets are not only ineffective, they're counterproductive. You no longer have to be prey to unscrupulous diet companies and their false claims of lasting success. You can stop the diet-to-diet seesaw now. Instead, you can discover what's really driving your urge to overeat and to carry extra weight, and you can learn what it is that you really need in order to be free of your food addiction and become healthy in body, mind, and spirit.

2

THE PURSUIT OF TRUE HAPPINESS, AND THE END OF ADDICTION

In talking about compulsive eating and why diets can never work, I think it's important to first address a more general problem in our society—one that I believe is the most important factor responsible for the epidemic of obesity and eating disorders today: the problem of how unhappy we've become. We seem to have moved further and further away from happiness by eschewing the real and true and pursuing the false. Instead of seeing the value of people and things of substance, we've become seduced by the flashy and the superficial. It's like we've all turned away from bread and butter and are trying to live on candy. Not only does it leave us malnourished, but it gives us a stomachache and rots our teeth.

To use another analogy, there's a road that leads to happiness and fulfillment, but few of us are taking it. Many of us are racing toward these goals with all the energy we can muster, but we're on the wrong path. If some of us happen upon the road, we don't recognize it for what it is and get off as soon as we've gotten on. There's a reason why we're lost and a reason we keep on running down the wrong road. I believe that once we see where we've erred, we'll be able to get ourselves onto the right road and stay on it, but this involves effort.

The good news is that most of us are not that far off-track in our search for happiness. We're just misguided. We're products of our families, society, and culture, and we've grown up learning lessons from all these sources about how to achieve this elusive goal. We might know people who are truly happy. We might also know people who seem to have all the right trappings, and we mistakenly think they're happy, too. Understanding this difference will be very helpful in our own process of discovery.

Where have we gone wrong? That's a whole book in itself. Suffice it to say that we've gotten into the habit of confusing a spiritual state—happiness—with a material state—the possession of commodities. By spiritual, I mean that which is related to our inner life. Happiness is the indescribable, powerful state we experience when we love, worship, or pray, are at peace, feel fulfilled, enjoy nature, create, or are playful. It's something that resides in the heart and soul. Whatever you imagine the soul is it's the domain of love and happiness.

Today, we try to find happiness by going after "candy," that is, accumulating things like money, power, acquaintances, objects, influence, or fame. We take on bad habits like overeating, smoking, drinking, gambling, shopping, bed hopping, or drug use in the hope that these, too, will lead us to happiness. We North Americans indulge freely in all of these but they haven't brought us happiness. On the contrary, we're less and less happy the more we have, because we're focusing our time and energy away from the "bread-and-butter" things that would give us real fulfillment, meaning, satisfaction, and inner peace.

In our increasing desperation for pleasure, we're increasingly less able to appreciate something or someone for its own qualities and instead we've begun to view people and things as interchangeable objects for our personal consumption. It's like we're these giant babies, lumbering about with wide-open mouths, but no matter how much "candy"—in the form of junk food, tech toys, designer drugs, dollars, or conquests—we cram down our insatiable throats, we can't be satisfied. We've become bottomless pits of need, wanting and having more yet feeling ever hungrier and more frustrated, because none of these things can ever make us happy.

If you were to look at the so-called happy people in your life, they might be the ones with all the candy: they've accumulated all the objects, fans, and bad habits. On the other hand, they have no sense of purpose or self and are constantly dealing with the problems associated with unconscious overindulgence. If you look at the truly happy, they're those who prefer bread and butter: they're connected with others, at home in their environment, and alive and whole within themselves. Real happiness comes not from all that candy, but from substantial things like meaning, purpose, and connection.

Many of us know this at some level but that knowledge hasn't encouraged us to look for nonmaterial types of happiness. We've become spiritually lazy. At this time in history, things have gotten too easy and convenient for us; we've gotten used to touching a button and expecting an automatic and effortless payoff. We've come to expect, even demand, that everything be "quick and easy," "instant," "painless," "guaranteed," and even "virtual."

The problem is it's the "guaranteed" loans and "quick and easy" investments that have robbed people of their life savings in Ponzi schemes and gotten our economy in the crisis it's in. We're eating "instant" foods that lack the flavor, texture or nutritional value of the real thing. Our virtual relationships are depriving us of the last shreds of intimacy, further undermining the integrity of the family. Our obsession with things being "painless" is creating a society of people numb to all but the most intense, violent, or perverse of experiences. And none of it has anything to do with happiness.

So what does? That's where the paradox lies. It's not in our endless consumption of resources, commodities, money, and even each other or in overindulging in risky substances or activities. It's definitely not in trying to anesthetize ourselves from anything uncomfortable and then overcompensating by subjecting ourselves to brutal horror films, violent video games, or bizarre, devoid-of-intimacy representations of sexuality online. It's in coming back to the bread-and-butter basics and recognizing that happiness is simplicity itself. It comes from reclaiming our nature as sensitive, caring beings that are an integral part of life on this planet.

The so-called American dream is a bust, and it's evidenced in the state of things right at this moment. The epidemic of obesity, the crisis in the banks and stock market, the pervasive lack of manners, the rising crime rates, and the anger, disenfranchisement, jealousy, greed, and hatred people feel toward one another in a continent of freedom and plenty are all indications that things have gone awry. The more we try to fill the spiritual void within ourselves with materialistic solutions, the more empty and unhappy we are, and the more hopeless and enraged we'll become. We're burning ourselves out pursuing this false dream, leaving us little energy with which to look for something real.

Rather than lashing out at one another, giving up in despair, indulging in meaningless pursuits, or trying like greedy children to take all the candy for ourselves, there's another option. We can stop the vicious circle of wasted energy and suffering now and put our attention toward achieving real and lasting rewards. *Not more stuff but more joy.* We can put our energy toward freeing ourselves from the prison we're trapped in, that's created by our unending consumption, addictions, and exploitation of people and things.

In our pursuit of pleasure through materialism, we've lost touch with who we really are. We've become preoccupied with external measures of fulfillment when it's always been something that dwells within us. One of our problems is that we don't always feel entitled to go after happiness directly, so we find ourselves "cheating" and looking for it in odd places. We'll buy new shoes or have a chocolate bar or a drink to reward or soothe ourselves after a hard day. It's because we're ambivalent about looking inward and asking ourselves directly, "what do I really need in order to be happy?"

Some of the critical messages we grew up hearing from our families and from society have gotten us confused about the pursuit of happiness. We mistake this pursuit for self-indulgence, egocentrism, or greed, but it's nothing like these things. In fact, truly happy people are the most generous, altruistic people around because they're so fulfilled that their joy overflows effortlessly. It's not wrong to look for happiness as long as we do it with a conscious awareness that hurting, exploiting, or stealing from others will take us in the opposite direction.

Some people feel guilty about pursuing happiness when there's so much unhappiness in the world. They think, "how could I be so selfish when others are suffering?" The answer to this is that *happiness begets more happiness,* and the happier you are, the more it will spread. The pursuit of real happiness, by definition, involves creating positive energy in the world. If the people close to you are happy it will spread to you, and if you're happy the people around you will become happier, recycling the happiness back to you. Still, someone has to start the cycle or there won't be any happiness to share.

Excitement, drama, or stimulation can be mistaken for happiness but these are the candy. Those of us who've become numb to our own feelings need to be overstimulated just to feel alive, never mind happy. If, instead, we rediscover our human capacity for sensitivity and take the time to tune in to our own and others' needs and feelings, then happiness is possible. Instead of requiring ever more intense sensations, we can appreciate the subtleties of simple, bread-and-butter things like a smile, the sun's warmth, the song of a bird, or a warm hug.

When it comes to consuming as a means to happiness, be it food or anything else, we have to understand that no matter how much we take in, it'll never be enough. Eating is assuredly a pleasurable activity, but in itself, can never be the major source of someone's happiness. Anything pleasurable is good in moderation. In excess, pleasure becomes a source of suffering as the consequences for our overindulgence begin to accrue. Do we really need to supersize all our meals and snacks?

When it comes to eating, the consequences of excess can be weight gain and medical problems such as diabetes, high blood pressure, and heart disease. There are also feelings of remorse, shame, and self-reproach tied to overindulgence. Also, since pleasure alone isn't ultimately satisfying, it's easy to get caught up in pursuing more and more of it in the incorrect belief that eventually, the pleasure will turn into happiness. The pursuit of pleasure is a dead end, because happiness comes from a state of freedom, not from endless need.

Life can be painful. It's filled with challenges and sacrifices and can sometimes seem brutal and overwhelming, especially to a child. Many of us grow up holding on to our childlike perspective in certain areas of our lives so that often, the normal adult difficulties we're facing seem unbearable. As a result, many of us shut ourselves down emotionally, thinking that this is the best way to cope. Unfortunately, it's the opposite of what we need to do in the face of challenges.

Shutting ourselves down emotionally deprives us of important information we'd otherwise gain by being responsive to our own needs and to the people and things in our environment. Lacking this information, we're unable to make the kinds of choices that would lead to happiness. Being numb also makes it difficult to empathize with others, so it's easier to be insensitive or hurtful toward them. Making other people unhappy can only lead to our unhappiness, because their hurt or sadness makes them unable to behave in a loving or positive way toward us or in the world.

A big part of happiness comes from self-acceptance. Accepting who you are creates an easier and less stressful existence. Self-acceptance isn't the same as an attitude of complacency or irresponsibility. It means loving yourself enough to want to be the best you can be. Self-acceptance doesn't lead to smugness or self-satisfaction but to personal growth, because it's the most fertile ground for positive change. While self-hatred creates despondency and hopelessness, making it impossible to change anything about yourself, self-love gives you energy and motivates you to develop further as an individual and to maximize your potential.

Some people think that the way to be happy is by "having it all," but I strongly disagree. Once you have it all, what's there to live for? Also, what if "having it all" doesn't do the trick? What if it's a big disappointment? Or, what if it means that you now have to juggle too many balls at once? Then it's like owning the proverbial white elephant, which is supposed to be a great prize, but is really a terrible burden.

I think it's better to start by being content with what you have. Not that you shouldn't want a better life, but you can learn to appreciate all that you have now. This is not settling, because if you feel that something is missing, you can strive for that. Some people always want more and are never satisfied with what they have. These folks are deeply frustrated and constantly running after the next thing, and the next, in the false hope that it will finally be enough.

We, as a society, need to know that in life, more isn't better, and that it's not always possible to get everything we want, the way we want it. You have to be flexible about what's actually available to you and learn to let go of what you can't have, while enjoying what you do have. Otherwise, you'll never achieve happiness.

Creativity fosters happiness, because being creative is something you can do all by yourself, for yourself, and is something meaningful that you can share with others. It's wonderful to feel that you can make something, build something, or solve a problem on your own. It gives you a sense of empowerment and the knowledge that you're self-sufficient. There's nothing like knowing that you can generate something beautiful or useful that causes pleasure or benefits the world. Creativity can also be done collaboratively, in which the best in each person is brought out in pursuing the project.

Generosity and altruism also bring happiness, because true generosity comes from an open heart and causes the heart to open further. This opening makes more room in the heart, allowing more love and positive energy to fill you. Being open hearted is the source of empathy. We feel connected to others by understanding their struggles, and we take pleasure in the gifts we share with others. Whereas giving from a sense of obligation creates feelings of disconnectedness, deprivation, and even resentment, giving from a heart overflowing with loving kindness leads to the experience of joy and a deeper sense of belonging.

Some people think that happiness comes from being admired, feared, or obeyed. They think that they'll be happy by being on top. These are actually very sad people whose so-called happiness comes from bullying, oppressing, or exploiting others and feeling superior to those they've subjugated. Dominating others can't possibly bring happiness, because there will always be those who are independent of this control, those who have more, or those who are superior themselves.

It's a no-win situation, because happiness based on a power struggle or competition is happiness dependent on other people. The power to be happy has to come from within or it can easily be taken away. It's paradoxical: those who try to dominate or compete with others have no hold on their own happiness, whereas those who are kind and generous have a never ending, internal source of happiness. People who have the power to improve their own lives and the lives of others are a lot happier than people who try to have power over others.

Happiness isn't something that comes for free. It takes work, but is well worth it. Our society promotes the idea of the "free ride," where work isn't necessary for achieving your goals. The easier something is to obtain, the better it's said to be, but this is a falsehood. The best example of this is winning the lottery. Studies have shown that the majority of winners are worse off, financially and emotionally, than they were prior to winning.

It's not an issue of morality, where hard work is seen as virtuous. It's just that in reality, happiness doesn't simply fall into your lap. You almost always have to work for it. Sometimes you even have to make sacrifices for it. The years I spent in premed, med school, and then internship and residency were a worthwhile sacrifice. If I'd thought, "oh, it's too hard to do all that training," I'm sure that I wouldn't have found the satisfaction I experience every day doing what I love. Temporarily giving up your social life and perhaps even your career in order to raise children is another type of sacrifice, but one that brings great happiness as well.

Of course, hard work and sacrifice for the wrong reasons won't bring happiness. Exhausting yourself trying to do something you're not suited for is a waste of energy and will create frustration, not happiness. You must figure out where your talents lie and work on developing these particular abilities. You'll have a much better chance at success and happiness if you also understand where not to focus your energy.

Good things do take work, whether it's a relationship that requires commitment, compromise, and communication; a garden that needs tending; an educational program that requires long hours of study; or the practice required for developing a skill such as piano playing, tennis, or welding. Happiness comes when you've built a connection, learned something new, or feel empowered from mastering a new task. Happiness comes out of the satisfaction of putting effort and time into something and seeing it pay off. When things come too easily they're harder to appreciate, but the effort makes the reward that much sweeter.

One of the deepest types of happiness comes from a sense of being connected to and coresponsible for all living things. Exploiting or harming others for your gratification, taking things from others, or depleting the planet's resources is possible only if you don't care about anything but yourself. That's a very lonely place to live and can't possibly bring you happiness.

When you become empowered as an adult and connect to others out of choice, not need, you can start enjoying people rather than using them to heal your wounds or to fill a void in your life. Being empowered, your generosity comes not from a secret wish to get something in return but from an overflowing of loving-kindness. Knowing that you have the ability to make others happier will bring you greater happiness. There's joy in providing yourself or your family with the basic needs, but the happiness of participating in the good of the planet is altogether grander.

This doesn't mean that you must go out and become a social activist, but that you simply become aware that you don't exist in a vacuum and that your actions and choices affect everyone and everything. If you choose to recycle paper and plastic, turn off the tap as you're brushing your teeth, use nontoxic household cleaners, or eat organic food, these acts have enormously positive global ramifications. If we all help our neighbors, neuter our pets, mentor our youth, and take public transportation sometimes, we're changing the world for the better and are creating more happiness for everyone. It's a very different model than that of consuming as much as possible and competing with each other for resources. This way, you see that helping others do well has a positive impact on your well-being.

Happiness is most possible when you take responsibility for yourself and your choices. If you see the things that are happening in your life as random events or the fault of other people, then you have no power to change things. If you recognize that the common denominator in the challenges you face is always you, then you learn to make different choices that could lead to greater happiness. Of course, random bad things will always happen but even then, the way you respond to those situations can make the difference between happiness and suffering.

Happiness is only possible if you're firmly grounded in reality, as opposed to living in denial of what's going on around you or happening to you. There are many ways of not living in reality. For example, you could ignore a suspicious lump that turns out to be cancerous; you could be denying that your spouse's increasingly contemptuous and controlling behavior is an indication that he's become abusive, or you could be denying that his long, unexplained absences and refusal of intimacy are most likely signs of infidelity.

If you're not living in reality, you might be refusing to acknowledge certain indications from your boss that he's about to let you go; you might be telling yourself that your frequent chest pains are "just stress;" you could lending your hard-earned money to the gambling-addict friend who keeps promising and failing to pay it back or telling yourself that this next bowl of ice cream will finally make you feel better.

All these denials will inevitably lead to a terrible shock or worse, unless you wake up and take stock of what's really going on. There's no benefit to hopeful fantasy or magical thinking—the act of believing that things are the way you wish them to be. You're at a great disadvantage when you indulge in these things, because you have no power to affect reality or make changes for the better.

While in denial, you won't leave the abusive or unfaithful spouse, and might instead suffer humiliation, a beating, or worse. In a state of wishful thinking, you won't be able to improve your performance at work or begin to look for a different job, and could find yourself suddenly unemployed. Living in hopeful fantasy, you could end up with a heart attack when instead you could have embarked on a plan to improve your health. Rather than indulging in the false hope that a friend who keeps borrowing money is trustworthy, you could have invested your money in something that would have paid you dividends, rather than losing funds and friendship because of this person's gambling addiction. Finally, you can look at your food cravings, recognizing that no amount of sugar could sweeten your life and that your problems must be solved in a different way.

Just as happiness won't come if you can't be content with what you have and who you are, it's equally impossible if it's dependent on you changing the people you're with. It will only create conflicts and frustration if you try to force a friend or loved one to go against his desires or true nature. Certain behaviors are changed easily enough, but some things will never change. You can tell a person how you feel about their troubling behavior and then see whether it's something he's willing or able to change. If not, you need to ask yourself, "can I live with it?" If so, then you must stop trying to change him. If you can't, then you might have to walk away.

By the same token, you can't try to be someone different to please another person. Not being true to yourself can't lead to being happy, even if the false front you're presenting pleases the other person. If you're not authentic, you'll end up feeling alienated from yourself and from the other person, as the love they're giving will be for your persona, not for your true self. That's not to say you can't compromise and accommodate some of the other person's needs. You shouldn't try to fundamentally change who you are or expect it of others.

You can't depend solely on the love or approval of others to make you happy. You have to love yourself. Without self-love, you wouldn't feel fully entitled to be loved by others, and you wouldn't carry yourself in a way that lets people know that you feel deserving of their love. Loving yourself, giving love to others, and receiving love create a positive flow of energy that leads to happiness.

Trying to get someone to heal your pain, build your self-esteem, or take away your loneliness is something that will only lead to unhappiness and resentment. Despite the fact that they might love you, another person can't give you self-worth, fix your loneliness, or soothe your pain. Loneliness, suffering, and insecurity are part of the human condition and each one of us is responsible to deal with these things on our own.

Happiness comes from a combination of self-love and real love from others, not from trying to get others to love you by being "nice" or "helpful." If you please in order to get love, the person isn't responding to who you really are but to the fact that your behavior is pleasing. You'll always wonder whether he likes you for your ingratiating behavior or for your true self.

One of the paradoxes of happiness is that *in order to be happy, first you have to be sad.* Let me explain: as you grow up, you'll experience losses or disappointments. Whether or not your parents were caring and loving, childhood inevitably brings its share of hurts and frustrations due to illness or addiction, death or divorce, financial difficulties, social or political strife.

Whatever you lived through as a child, you need to deal with your losses as an adult if you're going to be happy. You have to take a good look at your past and face the truth about any hurts or disappointments. Then, by consciously grieving your losses, you'll be able to let go of any residual sadness, pain, or anger you might have been carrying with you into the present day. You'll emerge from the grieving process with a clean slate and will no longer be burdened by any residual pain. It's not easy to revisit the painful past, but not doing so could allow the emotional wounds of childhood to interfere with the full experience of happiness today.

Happiness comes from the experience of freedom. It's not possible for someone enslaved or imprisoned to be truly happy. There are many types of slavery and many prisons in which you could be trapped. You can be a slave to mistaken beliefs about yourself and the world or enslaved by an addiction such as compulsive eating, shopping, gambling, or drug use. You can be trapped in a dysfunctional relationship or a prisoner of your obsession with food, weight, and dieting. Without freedom there's much suffering, so it's imperative that you work on correcting erroneous beliefs, healing compulsive behaviors and letting go of obsessive thinking patterns.

Happiness comes from living in the present. If you're looking ahead to the future too much and daydreaming about how you wish things were, you can't be happy now. If you're dwelling on the past (as opposed to looking back in order to deal with unfinished business); if you're berating yourself for old mistakes or carrying a grudge against someone who hurt you, you can't be happy now. You need to stop trying to leap forward or backward; all you have is right now. If things aren't the way you want them to be today, it's your responsibility to change them for the better. Fantasizing will waste time you could be spending on improving your life in this moment.

One important element necessary for happiness is flexibility. Being flexible and adaptable is a biological survival mechanism. Species have survived or perished based on their ability or inability to adapt to changing environments. You need to be flexible in your thinking, because intellectual rigidity creates a barrier to learning. If you can't learn from your mistakes, you'll keep recreating the same difficulties. If, on the other hand, you're open minded and can see the different sides to each story, you'll be able to not only survive but also thrive. This mental flexibility will allow you to learn and change for the better— ingredients in a happy and successful life.

Emotional flexibility is equally important. You must know your feelings, express them, and then release them. Otherwise, the pressure of unexpressed feelings will build up inside you, and you'll end up with emotional leakage in the form of a snide remark to a loved one, a tearful breakdown at the office, or an angry outburst toward another driver on the road. These types of emotional leaks will always have negative repercussions.

Knowing how to receive is essential for happiness. Too many of us mistakenly believe that we should be able to do everything for ourselves and don't ask for help when we need it. It's important to be self-sufficient but it's also important to recognize that we're all interdependent. No one should feel that they can't ask for help or receive a favor or a compliment. When we're in trouble, refusing help only perpetuates our suffering and most likely hurts our loved ones, as well. Receiving from others not only is good for us but it allows the other person to take pleasure in being able to give. If no one was willing to receive, altruism would be impossible.

There are three basic adult tasks you'll need to master if you're going to be happy. They are: taking care of business, following the dream, and problem solving.

Taking care of business has two components. There's doing what's necessary, including the basic adult tasks, such as going to work, running your household, paying the bills and your taxes, and caring for loved ones. Then there's "doing the right thing," such as helping an elderly neighbor, caring for a sick friend, giving to charity, being politically active, or volunteering.

The second adult task—following the dream—includes getting in touch with your fondest dreams and going after them. It's true that there has to be a balance between what's practical and what you hope for, but if you give up every aspect of your dreams, it won't be possible to be happy. You may need to adjust your plans and be flexible about what's realistic to pursue. This flexibility, however, will allow for the possibility of new, perhaps better versions of your dreams.

The third adult task—problem solving—can also be separated into two parts. These are the problems that arise when random events happen, and the problems that we're totally or partially responsible for creating. In life, a lot of things just happen. Some are good, some are neutral, and some can be pretty bad. You can't control the random events of life, be they natural disasters, the loss of a loved one, illness, or economic downturns. What you can do is make responsible, mature choices about how you'll deal with these challenges.

The less angry, indignant, or helpless you feel about the bad things that happen in your life and the more you take responsibility for dealing with them, the better the outcome will be. Dealing with life's challenges will empower you and enable you to develop self-trust which will, in turn, improve your chances of making the next challenge an opportunity for growth and learning. Even from sad, painful, or scary events, happiness can grow.

The second aspect of problem solving involves the problems you create for yourself. Perhaps you're in the habit of choosing partners who are neglectful or abusive. Perhaps you're developing health problems due to binge eating. Maybe you have a lateness problem that's causing conflicts in the workplace, or it could be that speeding is putting you at risk of getting into an accident or losing your driver's license.

There are two factors you need to be aware of when dealing with self-created problems. The first is to recognize that there are real, unconscious reasons for these self-destructive or self-sabotaging behaviors. If you acknowledge and deal with the emotional issues that are causing you, for example, to binge on chips or ice cream in the evening, you'll be able to stop this behavior and eventually resolve the weight and health problems you've created.

The second thing to know is that being self-critical about having caused yourself problems only leads to further problems. Self-reproach doesn't motivate you to do better. It's preferable to develop an attitude toward yourself that I call "ruthless compassion," which I'll explain in detail later on. With a compassionate and understanding attitude, you'll be able to explore your unconscious motivations for creating these problems, work on fixing the current situation, and most likely prevent future difficulties.

With compassionate ruthlessness there's no "get out of jail free" card. It means taking responsibility for the consequences of your actions and making changes where necessary. You don't have to berate yourself for your mistakes, but you should not pretend that you didn't make them, either. By facing up to your misguided behaviors with ruthless compassion, you'll be able to break any vicious circle you've created. For example, you can break the cycle of overeating, cruel self-criticism, and further overeating to soothe the pain of this unrelenting self-criticism.

If you're engaging in the three basic adult tasks, you'll be well on the road to happiness because you won't have to deal with the fallout of neglecting life's basics. There won't be dishes piling up in the sink, interest to pay on back taxes, children running wild, or bill collectors calling. Instead of wasting time sorting out the mess you've created by neglecting the necessities, you'll have time to pursue real fulfillment. With the business taken care of, you're free to follow your dreams, and because these dreams are realistic, they're achievable.

In childhood, there are four factors essential for present and future happiness: physical security and comfort, emotional fulfillment, a proper education, and the absence of trauma.

First, it's necessary for a child to grow up in a safe, clean, stable, and peaceful environment. Interestingly, once the minimal levels of these physical necessities have been reached, this category ends up being the least important of the four, as I'll explain in a moment.

As well as the basic physical requirements, a growing child needs to be loved, acknowledged, valued, affirmed, understood, protected, and defended. These emotional necessities of early life enable a child to grow into a confident, successful adult who's capable of a high level of functionality in all areas. This is a much more important factor than the former, because if any of these needs are absent, the child will grow up with emotional problems or difficulties in one or more areas of functioning.

The third factor is a proper education. This means both an academic and emotional education, including learning how to function in the adult world and good values such as responsibility, kindness, and generosity. A child should learn about her right to respect and dignity, how to have healthy boundaries, and how to say "no." A child should learn that she has choices in life, and that these will have rewards and consequences. Education in childhood is more important than the physical necessities because without education, the child isn't equipped either practically or psychologically for adult life.

The last factor relates to childhood trauma. Abuse can come at the hands of parents or through not being protected by parents who, through neglect, denial, or being distracted with other things, allow the child to be abused by others. Trauma can include any type of severe shock, hurt, or loss. These terrible things can be mitigated by the presence of a strong and supportive family and community. In the absence of such support, childhood trauma and abuse can have long-lasting repercussions, including depression, anxiety, interpersonal and work difficulties, and various addictions.

Emotional support, love, protection from harm, an education that teaches good values, and self-respect are the most important factors for a child's future happiness. Once the basic physical necessities of life are present, children can get on with their lives. Little ones won't notice the lack of material objects. What they can't forego is the love, care, and affirmation of their parents and community and the tools to make it in the world—both practically and psychologically. Children need to grow up into adults who have self-esteem, self-confidence, resilience, a good attitude, and the ability to keep learning and growing. The presence of emotional nurturing, a good education, and the absence of trauma or abuse will provide them with what they need for future happiness.

In my early 20s, I began taking modern dance lessons with a professional company. The first move the teacher showed the new students was how to fall without getting hurt. It made a lot of sense to me because during practice, we were constantly changing direction, leaping, rolling, and throwing ourselves around. By teaching us how to fall, our teacher made it possible for us to fully participate in all of the dancing.

It's the same in most other aspects of life: you have to learn how to fall. One of my patients revealed to me that after she got hurt in love early in her life, she hadn't attempted another relationship. She also began avoiding close friendships. She never understood that she could survive getting hurt in romantic or platonic love. She never learned how to fall.

Learning how to tolerate hurt and loss is an essential survival tool, and therefore an essential ingredient in happiness. First, you have to know that falling is inevitable, so you won't be devastated if you happen to land on your backside. If you can fall and get up again, you can trust that the next time, it won't be so bad either. Also, you can reflect on what happened, and perhaps even prevent yourself from falling again. Being able to get through a painful time means not having to shut down emotionally or indulge in too much food, drink, or drugs in order to numb the pain. If you can fall and get right back up again, you can learn from your experiences and maybe even grow wiser.

In overcoming any addiction, you're going to have to attend to the needs of the child within: you must face, grieve and let go of the wounds of the past, give the child the love and comfort she desperately craves and silence the internalized parent whose pushy and critical messages only backfire (I'll discuss these three steps in greater detail later in the book). These steps which attend to the needs of the child within are essential but insufficient. If you want to be free of addiction, you must also meet your fundamental adult need for true happiness. When you feed your soul, you'll no longer need to feed your addiction.

On the road to happiness there are pitfalls, bumps, detours, and roadblocks. You'll fall down, and storms will come. You'll be tempted to get sidetracked, and sometimes you'll want to just sit down in the middle of the road and cry. Navigating all this is a natural part of the journey toward happiness. The lessons you learn through overcoming adversity, grieving your losses, healing from your hurts, helping others, and letting others help you are all part of the process.

Finally, here are a few of my thoughts on how to have more happiness:

Happiness is slow and steady. Joy bubbles up.

Happiness is paradoxical; let it find you.

Laugh a lot more.

Be brave or live with regret.

Say yes a lot more.

Do things that scare you a bit.

Don't take yourself too seriously.

Don't let pride get in the way of what your heart desires.

Be vulnerable, even if it means getting hurt.

Trust yourself.

Do more with a lightness of attitude.

Cultivate sensitivity.

Be curious.

Never underestimate the importance of good boundaries.

Have a good cry now and then.

Be strong, but not brittle.

Slow down to feel more and enjoy more.

Stay awake.

Live in the present.

Let yourself be moved.

Let people in.

Refuse to be imprisoned by hatred, jealousy, vengefulness, greed, arrogance, or self-pity.

Learn to receive with grace.

Practice listening. Tell those who care what you need.

Invest your energy wisely.

Stop wasting your time on people who don't deserve you.

Go for what you want instead of running from what you fear.

Feed your soul more and your belly less.

Be with people who bring out the best in you.

Be generous.

Play more.

Make things happen.

Forego drama.

Stop complaining.

3

FOOD AS THE FALSE SOLUTION: THE REAL CAUSE OF COMPULSIVE EATING

SUZIE'S STORY

One of the greatest successes in my practice was Suzie, a university student in her early 20s who was extremely overweight. She had come to therapy believing that she was from a "close, loving family," but soon it became clear that her mother was controlling and rejecting and her father was self-involved and neglectful. Eventually she realized that every time she visited them, she came away feeling deeply inadequate and frustrated that she still couldn't get them to give her some positive attention. This made her feel terrible about herself and always led to an episode of binge eating.

During her therapy, Suzie realized how destructive it was for her to spend time with her parents. She saw that she'd been using food to compensate for the love that she was missing and to soothe her feelings of emptiness and longing. These insights led her to separate from her parents, both emotionally and physically.

From that moment on, Suzie began to lose weight. She did so without dieting; in fact, she wasn't even thinking about eating or weight. When she no longer needed to soothe herself over the frustration associated with her parents, the urge to overeat disappeared. Seventy-five pounds gradually came off over a year. In her therapy, Suzie had done the difficult work of seeing the truth about her parents and healing her pain, which meant that she didn't have to work at losing weight.

It's been more than seven years, and Suzie has kept the weight off. More importantly, her self-esteem has improved tremendously and as a result, she's gotten a much better job, a better apartment, and several new friends. She's even in her first serious relationship. None of this would have been possible if she'd continued to deny how much her ongoing relationship with her parents was keeping her unhappy and making her overeat.

As I said before, compulsive eating is to a great extent a response to emotional wounds and needs. The wounding occurs in childhood as a result of inadequate or hurtful parenting, as well as other hurts or losses encountered during childhood. Fortunately, you don't need perfect parents to grow up without emotional wounds. As I explained previously, you just need parents who're able to love and care for you, provide you with the necessary education, and protect you from abuse. It's the presence or absence of their emotional wounds that makes the difference between adequate and inadequate parents.

In general, if you were lucky enough to have had good enough parents, your emotional wounds will likely be minimal and any eating problem you have won't be severe. You might not even have much of a weight problem. On the other hand, those with more serious eating and weight problems will more than likely have been raised by parents who had a greater degree of emotional wounds. It wasn't necessarily deliberate on your parents' part, but they were unable or unwilling to meet your basic childhood needs.

Not everyone who's been emotionally wounded will have an eating problem. Some people will have symptoms of anxiety or depression. Some might have other addictions or experience difficulties in their relationships or at work. Emotional wounds can show up in many different areas of a person's life, but for the purposes of this book, we'll focus on how being wounded can contribute to the problems of compulsive eating and being overweight.

Parents don't have to be deliberately hurtful or neglectful to cause their children emotional wounds. They could care about you and mean well, but if they haven't faced and dealt with their own emotional issues, then it's inevitable that they're going to pass on these wounds—great or small—to you. It's your parents' responsibility, whatever they experienced in their own childhoods, to discover and resolve their own emotional issues prior to starting a family.

There are many different types of parents responsible for creating problems in their children. Some parents are so wounded that they're not up to the task of parenting. They get so overwhelmed that they let their children basically raise themselves. Others are caring but inadequate. They entered into parenthood with low self-esteem and model this poor self-image to their children. Some parents are rejecting. They regard their children as a "burden," who they resent. Some are so deeply wounded that they're filled with hatred, greed, or rage. They need to control and dominate other people (including their children), who they see as objects to exploit for their own gratification.

There are parents who are caught up in situations that have made it difficult or impossible for them to connect with their children. This type of parent has a good heart, but is distracted by things that challenge his or her ability to be available to his or her children. You could call this style of parenting detached. Some parents are overly perfectionist and unreasonably expect an adult level of competence at tasks their child is only beginning to learn. Some parents are unable to empathize with their children and can be extremely hard-hearted toward them. Some make their child responsible for the emotional well-being of the parent. This is beyond a child's capabilities and therefore causes the child to feel guilty and inadequate. There are parents who resent their children for their promise, beauty, talent, or intelligence. Rather than wanting their child to do better than they did, these parents are competitive and may even try to thwart their child's success.

All of these different types of parents cause their children varying degrees of distress. Growing up with any of the parents described previously could cause someone to have low self-esteem, to be insecure or inadequate, to feel hurt, angry, or undeserving of love or success. The child could grow up full of anxiety and with powerful feelings of helplessness. They could be struggling with shame and worthlessness, feeling lonely and empty, and turning to food as a comfort. There can be feelings of frustration, resentment, and guilt, as well as a deep need for love, but ambivalence about it because they've been led to believe that they don't deserve it. The child could grow up with lot of confusion. All of these things can predispose someone to overeat in the attempt to find healing, soothing, and nurturing in food.

It's certainly not always necessary to stop seeing your parents to heal the wounds they caused you, especially if they meant well and hurt you inadvertently. Sometimes, your wounds had more to do with painful circumstances, such as poverty, the illness of a sibling, or the death of a loved one. In Suzie's case, her parents were an extreme example of bad parenting and could be described as "toxic." When it comes to toxic parents, it is necessary to separate from them because being in their presence literally will make you sick.

As I mentioned previously, the internalized parent derives from your actual parents, guardians, or society at large. All the direct and indirect messages you absorbed during childhood are distilled into the voice of your internalized parent. If this inner voice is harsh or judgmental, it's because your actual parents or parent figures were this way. If you were made to feel inadequate, guilty, or ashamed, the internalized parent will reiterate these messages in your head. Whether or not your parents did this intentionally, all the less-than-positive messages entered your unconscious mind and consolidated into the internalized parent.

If this voice tells you that you "should" do something, it's because your parent figures gave you this idea. If the voice tells you that you're not lovable, it's because your parents either weren't able to give you enough love or modeled their lack of self-love to you. If the internalized parent criticizes you for something, it's because your parents or parent-figures let you know, directly or indirectly, that it was "bad," and if this voice makes you feel guilty or ashamed, it's because you were made to feel this way as a child, whether deliberately or inadvertently.

Unfortunately, rather than being your conscience (what some people erroneously believe is the function of the internalized parent), it's mainly a bully and tormentor. It makes you feel bad about yourself and rubs salt in your emotional wounds. You might think it exists to motivate you or to keep you "on the straight and narrow," but really, its role is just to dominate and oppress you.

Why would we have such a negative voice in our heads? Perhaps it's a primitive protective mechanism that has simply gone awry. Perhaps our developing psyche has no capacity to compensate for inadequate or hurtful parenting.

Whatever the reason, the internalized parent is completely unnecessary for normal adult functioning. We can eliminate it without any adverse effects: an adult doesn't need a parent to tell her what to do or how to think.

This inner voice of negativity can be mildly critical: the "inner critic." It can be cruel: the "inner opponent." Sometimes, this voice is extremely destructive: the "inner killer," which causes self-hatred, emotional paralysis, and self-sabotage. In the case of self-hatred, it's the internalized parent hating the child within. In self-love, however, it's the adult self-loving the child within. As an adult, our positive self-regard is between the adult and the child within, while our negative self-regard comes from the hostility of the internalized parent toward the child.

Facing the truth about your parents isn't easy, but it will not only enable you to heal your emotional wounds, but also prevent the next generation from being wounded in the same way. Like I said before, if your parents hurt you or were unable to meet your needs, it's because of inadequate love or care from their parent-figures or because they grew up in a family or society that caused them to be wounded.

Let's say that your parents were unable or unwilling to attend to their own wounds. If so, they were doomed to pass the wounds on to you despite their best intentions. You might not want to think badly of them—and you don't have to—but if you can't see how they've wounded you, you won't be able to heal. This means that you must understand how wounds keep being passed down through the generations until they're finally addressed. If you face the truth today about your wounded and wounding parents, the pattern will stop with you. It may be uncomfortable to see your parents in this light but it's the only way for you to heal and to prevent your wounds from being passed on to your children.

You might be someone who feels so loyal to your parents that you would never dream of connecting them to your current problems. You might say to yourself, "they did the best they could." This may be true but it doesn't negate the fact that, regardless of their intentions, your parents' actions or inaction had a negative impact on you. What matters is not whether they *did their best* but whether what they did was *best for you.* If your loyalty to your parents interferes with your ability to be happy and successful, just ask yourself this: would "good enough" parents want you to put sparing their feelings ahead of your own emotional healing?

We all need parents who love and protect us and give us what we need in order to grow up happy, healthy, and whole. If you've received "good enough" parenting, you're more likely to grow up to be confident, high-functioning, and free of emotional problems or addictions. In the absence of such parenting or when there have been other losses or traumas, the child within remains at the forefront of the personality as it seeks emotional healing and compensation for its wounds through overeating or other addictions.

Children take everything personally so it's natural to interpret a lack of love or the experience of trauma or abuse as something you must have deserved.

EMOTIONAL OVEREATING

Recent Titles in
The Praeger Series on Contemporary Health and Living

The internalized parent reinforces this by telling the child within that how you were treated by your parents was due to your being unlovable, unworthy, or defective. Sadly, a child can't understand that parents don't give children what they "deserve," but rather, what the parents are *capable* of giving. While it's true that parents respond to some extent to their children's needs and personalities, the hurtful things that happened in your childhood had nothing to do with your behavior or qualities, and everything to do with your parents' limitations.

In truth, being wounded doesn't necessarily make a person unable to love. It's a bit of a mystery why some very deeply wounded individuals can still love others, while some less-wounded ones can't. I suppose that some people are simply more susceptible to having their hearts shut down as a result of their wounds.

All living beings are by nature lovable, and no one needs to *do* anything in order to be loved. You only need to be with those people who are *able to love you*. If a child tries to be "good" and *earn* love, it will be a waste of his energy. Whether in childhood or as an adult, if you try to *get* others to love you and they aren't able to, you could end up soothing your hurt feelings by overeating. If you see that your parents' behavior toward you wasn't a reaction to your being inadequate or unlovable, then you won't need to try so hard to please others or to overfill your belly to soothe your heart.

Suzie had wanted to believe that her parents loved her, as most of us do. It's awful to imagine that your parents didn't love you the way you needed to be loved. Suzie had been tolerating her parents' hurtful behavior, wanting to believe that she belonged to a close-knit family and hoping that one day, she'd feel truly loved. Through our work together, Suzie learned that she'd be able to heal her wounds without needing her parents to treat her differently. She came to understand that overcoming her compulsive eating had nothing to do with getting her parents to change. She learned tools for getting over the loss of parental love and care, and began to move on with her life.

Your childhood experiences of loss and pain might have led you to choose overeating as a solution but you don't have to dwell on past traumas in order to overcome them. Otherwise, you'd forever identify yourself as a victim. Blaming others for your problems is what children do, because they have no power to change their lives. It's preferable to be an empowered adult, as opposed to an "adult child" of hurtful parents, a "survivor" of abuse or someone "in recovery" from addiction.

Being an adult is about becoming independent from your parents and no longer living in reaction to them. It's seeing how they've affected you, dealing with whatever emotional wounds they might have passed on to you and then getting on with your life. Blaming your parents is living your life trapped in the past and abdicating responsibility for the problems you're facing. There can be no happiness without personal accountability. Seeing the truth about your parents is only a first step. The ultimate aim is to let go of the wounds they (deliberately, neglectfully, or inadvertently) caused you, any hurt or anger you feel toward them, as well as your dependence on them so that you can be free of your addictive behaviors.

As I said before, compulsive eating and all other addictions come, in large part, from the misguided attempts of the child part of the psyche to find love and nurturing and to heal her wounds. The needy, wounded child stays at the forefront of the psyche because her agenda takes precedence. The child within ought to be a background figure in the psyche of an adult, but unmet needs and unhealed emotional wounds prevent the child within from taking on its proper role as a minor aspect of the adult psyche. This, in turn, prevents you as an adult from pursuing the things that would bring you true happiness and fulfillment.

The internalized parent is overrepresented as well in this scenario because it follows that poor or inadequate parenting prevents the formation of a powerful adult identity and allows the internalized parent to dominate the psyche. In the absence of adequate parenting, the child fails to grow into a confident, competent adult who no longer needs a parent to guide, protect or nurture her. In such cases, the adult identity isn't strong enough to wrest control from the internalized parent. In the absence of a strong adult mediator, the child and parent parts of the psyche coexist in a constant state of conflict. This creates a vicious circle, making it tremendously difficult for the adult aspect to take charge and go about meeting her true needs.

When a person has grown up with inadequate or abusive parenting, they won't always demonstrate expected rational, reasonable adult behavior. What will emerge, instead, are the impulsive, irrational, despairing or rebellious behaviors of the child within. To the extent that the internalized parent is in charge at a given moment, the child will cooperate with the parental agenda. Eventually, though, the child gets angry enough at being criticized and controlled, or is overcome by such despair that she defies the internalized parent or ignores it. The child within, being the original self, has final veto power in the psyche over the admonitions of the internalized parent. Sadly, she doesn't have the mental sophistication to use this power to her best advantage.

The child within is the part of the psyche that holds all the feelings, attitudes, beliefs, and attributes you had as a child. If your childhood was "good enough," the child within exists to add passion, spontaneity, curiosity, and creativity to your existence. If, on the other hand, your childhood was lacking or hurtful, the child within is overly prominent in the psyche and all her childish attributes, such as impulsivity, selfishness, impatience, short sightedness, and poor judgment are front and center.

The child within, like all children, goes after quick and easy solutions. Addictions such as overeating are obvious choices for the child within because they appear to provide immediate gratification of her needs. For example, if the child is upset, scared, or angry, she can immediately soothe or numb herself with comforting food. The child isn't capable of recognizing that it actually doesn't feel as good as she thought it would, nor is she able to associate her choices with their natural consequences. The child doesn't associate weight gain with overeating, so this consequence doesn't deter her from continuing with the behavior.

While the child within is so preoccupied with looking for nurturing and healing, the adult identity can't come to the forefront of the psyche. As a result, there's no adult available to make rational choices about eating and weight, or to seek the things that will bring real fulfillment. The child is predominant because her need for healing and nurturing is a survival instinct and therefore the number one psychological priority. Because it's the child's nature to be stubborn, she persists in pursuing her ineffective strategy.

The child within maintains what I call *pathological hope*—the hope that she'll achieve what she wants, even when reality keeps showing her that she won't. Pathological hope isn't reality based; it's an incorrect belief that what's wished for will come true. It's one of the defining characteristics of the child within and it's what causes the child to keep on overeating and never give up in the absence of tangible success.

The child thinks, "if I eat just one more bowl of ice cream, then I'll finally be satisfied." When it doesn't work, she keeps on eating in the hope that eventually, healing will come. This is what makes the eating a compulsive behavior: the child is *compelled* to keep trying to get food to do the trick. She can't stop the behavior because her pathological hope spurs her on.

Those of you whose needs weren't met during childhood will have a poorly developed adult self. You may think that you're a fully fledged adult, but if you find yourself compulsively overeating, criticizing yourself for it, and then telling yourself that you should go on a diet, it means you have overdeveloped child and parent parts of the psyche and an underdeveloped adult identity. People grow into adulthood unaware that a wounded child within is calling the shots. Consciousness isn't an automatic function like breathing; it has to be practiced and developed. The adult self obviously needs to be your main identity when you've grown up, but when unhealed wounds fester inside, the adult is elbowed out by the overbearing internalized parent and the desperate, hopeful child. This is a bad situation, because only the adult part of you can become conscious of your emotional wounds and work to heal them.

It's only the adult self who can properly pursue the self-care, relationships, and goals that will meet your emotional needs and bring you true fulfillment. Until you become conscious that these three aspects of your psyche exist and are in conflict, it'll be impossible for the adult to take over as your predominant identity. It might also explain why often you find yourself pulled in different directions.

The term *cognitive dissonance* means that you find yourself doing things even when you know you shouldn't. Let's say that the child within is driving you to overeat as she pursues her illogical, hopeful agenda. The adult part wants to stop the binges, but it's underdeveloped, so you continue overeating. Cognitive dissonance is defined as "a lack of harmony in the mind."

If you have emotional wounds, the internalized parent vies with the child within for dominance in your psyche. The criticisms and "shoulds" you once heard as a child are now directed toward the child within. The internalized parent scolds the child, saying that she's bad for overeating; that she's "fat and disgusting."

Without outside assistance in becoming more conscious, the child part of the psyche is as unaware of the adult self as the adult is of the child. She doesn't realize that the adult is her ally and could make everything better if it were to take over as the primary identity and reject the negative inner messages, heal the child's wounds, and give her the love and soothing she never received. In this way, a strong adult identity could make overeating obsolete.

When the adult and child parts aren't connected through consciousness they can't cooperate, and you're powerless over your eating. When the adult and child within become aware of each other, your adult self can then assume the care of the child, the child can learn to trust the adult to heal her wounds and give her love, and you'll be able to eat as an empowered adult, free of compulsion or cognitive dissonance.

It's the hope of the child within that enough eating will eventually pay off, but it never will. The wounds of the past can't be healed by any addictive behavior. Overeating won't take away your hurt, anger, or shame; nor can it provide you with self-confidence or self-love. It won't replace anxiety or depression with happiness or silence the criticisms of the internalized parent. Your wounds can only be healed by your adult self. As long as the child is in charge, she'll look to external solutions like overeating, her wounds will remain unhealed, and the addiction will persist.

Developing a strong adult identity will enable everything to change: With a strong adult in charge, the child within will be able to let go of her pathological hope about eating and trust in the adult's ability to heal her wounds, protect her from the critic, and give her the love and care she's always needed. The adult can pursue meaningful work, relationships, and pastimes, instead of counterproductive addictions.

ISABELLA'S STORY

I remember Isabella, a pharmacist in her 30s, who shared how she could hear a three-way conversation in her head among the different parts of her psyche. One part (the child) said, "Oh, I want to eat this. I deserve it." Another part (the adult) responded, "You don't need to eat that. It's not food you're hungry for," and yet another part (the parent) said, "You disgusting loser! You have no self-control!"

Isabella's weak adult identity was caught between the pushy internalized parent who demanded that she diet and the hurt, needy child within who pursued immediate gratification. Her frequent binges meant that she was stuck in self-sabotage, which happens when the child within rejects or acts out against the internalized parent's messages.

As I said before, the adult self will develop normally if you had an adequate childhood. This environment provides the ingredients necessary for a strong adult identity: caring parents and other adults who *model* a strong, loving adult identity to the child who will then *internalize* the affirmation, care, and protection that she was given while growing up.

If you weren't raised under these ideal circumstances, you'll probably have difficulty in some of areas of adult functioning, depending on how bad things were for you and the degree of your natural resilience. You'll need to put some real work into becoming a fully fledged adult who's in touch with her needs and in charge of her behavior. This means making time to practice feeling and behaving like an adult and looking at things through adult eyes.

Good, adult functioning in some areas of your life doesn't mean you have a fully developed adult identity. It just means that not all of your choices and actions are driven by the child within. You shouldn't assume that if some aspects of your life, for example, your job or your creativity, are going well the child isn't in charge of other aspects, like eating and weight. You'll need to develop a more consistent adult identity to deal with your overeating and any other areas of difficulty you're experiencing.

The child self is a composite of all stages of your childhood, from birth to the beginning of adulthood, and contains all the feelings, memories, beliefs, expectations, joys, and traumas of your childhood. The child within is child-like, and therefore unable to take responsibility for her actions. Small and helpless, she's easily overwhelmed by people, situations, or emotions. Her moods are intense but rapidly changing.

The child within has little tolerance for anxiety or discomfort, and does whatever it takes to feel better as quickly and easily as possible. Because she lacks impulse control, she tends to act out her feelings rather than tolerating them internally. She's incapable of insight, so she's blind to her own behavior.

If your actions are being driven by the child within, you could go through life feeling and acting a lot like a child—whether or not you realize it. You could be so identified with the child that it wouldn't be possible for you to step outside yourself and look in on what the child is doing. The only way to get in touch with the child within and also identify the negative messages of the internalized parent is to fully inhabit the adult identity.

As I mentioned previously, the "inner killer" is a particularly vicious version of the internalized parent. This destructive force in the psyche takes on the sound of your own voice so it seems to be a part of you rather than an interloper. This is why you probably haven't been questioning the things it tells you, even when it torments you.

If you find yourself acting out with inappropriate anger toward people who are in positions of power, then most likely, the child's anger and frustration toward the inner critic are leaking from your unconscious mind into the real world. Your inner conflict is turning into outer conflicts with others and this acting out is going to cause you some problems.

Your resentment toward authority figures comes from the fact that unconsciously, they remind you of the critics you grew up with and the critical parental voice currently assaulting you. It's bad enough to have an inner conflict, but if you start to act out toward people who could fire you or have you put in jail, the parent-child conflict is creating a dangerous situation. For this reason alone, it's essential that you resolve your inner conflicts.

Being angry is a very uncomfortable emotional state for many people and especially for women. Society to some extent supports men in expressing their anger, but not so with women. Women will often repress their anger, not wanting to appear aggressive or hurtful. One way to repress anger is to stuff it down through eating. In this way, living with a constant inner conflict can potentially get you into trouble with other people, while also making you fat.

If you find yourself having difficulties functioning in one or more areas of your life, it could be because the child within is angrily "on strike" against the harshness of the inner critic. It could also be that she's feeling helpless and overwhelmed, and incapable of pleasing the critic. If you suffer from depression or anxiety, some of your symptoms might be related to the child's feelings of helplessness, hopelessness, or despair. Although the adult should be in charge of the psyche, it still needs the cooperation of the child within to get anything done. For this reason, the paralyzed child within makes everything you attempt a huge struggle, including any attempt to lose weight.

It's in a child's nature to see parental love and care as the solution to her wounds. If this was lacking, the child within is convinced that emotional healing will come not only from overeating or other addictions, but also from being nurtured by present-day love objects in the form of romantic partners or close friends. Unfortunately, the child within can't benefit from the love of other people. It's only the adult self who can love and heal her. Once you've grown into an adult, love coming from another person is wonderful but it can't be used by the child within to heal her wounds or meet her needs. Access to the child within is restricted to the adult self and the internalized parent.

The inner critic shames the child over her need for love and the way she's using relationships in the attempt to achieve her goals, and this parental scorn could then drive the child to turn once again to overeating. Conversely, your adult self can enjoy relationships for the companionship and romance they bring. The adult can validate the child's needs for love and healing and be the one to give her what she's seeking.

Our media represent our cultural norms. We're told, through the way women and girls are portrayed, that being extremely thin is most desirable. The child within reacts to these images with the same ambivalence she'd feel about any parental message. She'd initially want to please the parent, but would eventually give up in despair or act out in spite against the critic.

The more pressure there is to be very thin, whether from inner or outer "parents," the heavier some women will become. This is due to a child-induced backlash against unrelenting exhortations to be thinner. There's an epidemic of seesaw starving and overindulging that's evident in the extremes we're experiencing today: the starlets, singers, models, and even regular women who can, at least for a while, conform to the expectation of extreme thinness and the many, many women whose average size is increasing year by year.

Women in the skinny group have a few things in common: a very controlling inner critic and/or a very obedient child within who hopes to find love, approval, and healing by being extremely thin. In the overweight group, either the internalized parent isn't as controlling or the child within is less cooperative or more spiteful. It is no coincidence that we've witnessed so many previously skinny women eventually become heavy; the child within finally grew tired of working so hard to please the inner or outer critics. Eventually, the backlash hit them.

MARJORIE'S STORY

Marjorie, like so many of my patients, is a woman struggling with trauma from her childhood. Her father was verbally and physically abusive to her and her mother was passive and neglectful. She began overeating as a young girl, having observed her mother comfort herself with food. By the age of 10, she was already suffering from depression, in part because she was constantly being teased about her weight by a group of older children at school.

Marjorie, until lately, has been extremely overweight, having used food all these years to deal with her pain. The depression made her overeat to soothe herself and being heavy made her subject to taunting, which then made her eat more to numb her shame. She feels worthless and unlovable from not having been nurtured or protected by her parents, and helpless because of the years of bullying.

Before coming to therapy, Marjorie didn't understand why she couldn't stop eating, but now she's learned about the different parts of the psyche and how the child within is compelling her to overeat. She's been developing an adult identity and is working on healing her emotional wounds and giving herself the love and affirmation she never received. So far, she's lost 35 pounds and for the first time, she's filled with optimism about the possibility of overcoming this once-impossible problem.

As I said previously, emotional wounds can take many forms: They can emerge as sadness, anger, hurt, jealousy, or anxiety. They can be experienced as helplessness, frustration, guilt, shame, longing, loneliness, or inadequacy. Most of these emotions, because they're upsetting, will be buried in the unconscious; a part of your psyche you can't readily access.

These emotions stay buried because they arose at a time when you were young and helpless. Back then, any frightening, confusing, or upsetting experience seemed too overwhelming to bear. As a scared, helpless child, being in touch with your feelings was associated with going crazy, losing control, or even dying.

As a child, you also sensed that it could be dangerous to let your emotions out, either because you'd seem more vulnerable or because someone might get angry at you if you expressed an emotion of which they didn't approve. You might even have been terrified of the potentially destructive power of your emotions. If you observed a parent being violent or abusive, you'd have associated all powerful emotions with this destructiveness. In this way, you'd have become afraid that if you let out your feelings, you might hurt or even kill someone.

When you were young, psychological defense mechanisms (which exist to keep you safe, sane, and alive) kicked in when overwhelming emotions or needs arose within you. These mechanisms protect you from unbearably painful experiences by burying intolerable emotions, urges, and memories in the unconscious so that you could tolerate and survive the experiences. This is what is called an "adaptive response." It's the way a person instinctively adapts to an overwhelming, sanity-threatening, or life-threatening experience. Unfortunately, what's instinctive and adaptive when we're children becomes harmful—"maladaptive"—as we grow up.

The emotions or needs you couldn't tolerate when you were little are ones you're strong enough to deal with and must deal with now, because this is an essential part of the healing process. *Facing, grieving,* and *letting go* of the hurts and losses from your childhood will gradually diminish the pain of your emotional wounds, and when the pain diminishes, the child's need to deal with her wounds by overeating also decreases. These are an essential part of the process of overcoming any addiction; in fact, this process of facing, grieving, and letting go is the first task in what I call the "four-pronged approach" to healing addiction. (I'll discuss the other tasks shortly.)

Facing the truth of your past means that you look at what happened and acknowledge the reality of it without self-judgment. Facing your past means not telling yourself stories, making up explanations for why things were or justifying others' actions. If you can't see the truth, you won't be able to heal your wounds. It's not about blaming others for what's wrong in your life today but about understanding how the things that happened affected you so that you know what you need in order to heal.

Grieving involves allowing yourself to mourn your losses. These losses include anything you needed and didn't get as a child; anything that was taken away from you or that hurt you. Grieving will make it possible for you to release all the buried emotions inside through crying or finding a constructive outlet for your anger. It has nothing to do with confronting anyone with your hurt or angry feelings. It's not up to others to heal the child within you. It's about taking responsibility to unearth the feelings buried in your unconscious and finally let them out in a safe, healthy manner.

Grieving isn't wallowing in self-pity or self-indulgently feeling "wronged." It's not a sign of weakness to connect with your pain and cry. It takes courage to access these upsetting emotions and self-love to make the choice to free yourself from the pain you've lived with for so long. It's not bad to release your anger in a healthy way, either. In fact, releasing your anger will give you a sense of empowerment and relief.

Letting go follows naturally from the first two actions. Facing and grieving your losses will enable you to release the upsetting emotions that were stuck inside you. You'll be able to let go of your past and in this way, finally be free of your wounds. Whether your childhood had a few minor upsets or was very traumatic, these three actions will unburden you of any leftover emotional baggage. In this way, any compulsive behavior you've adopted in order to deal with these wounds can also be dropped.

Another important aspect of healing addiction is to combat the negativity coming from the internalized parent. (This is the second task of the four-pronged approach to healing addiction.) If your inner critic is still abusing the child within, it doesn't matter how much you grieve your losses, nurture the child within, or pursue your dreams. If the child is still being hurt by the internalized parent, she'll continue using food for the purpose of self-soothing.

The next two tasks required in overcoming compulsive eating (and any other addiction) are to give yourself what you really need. These include the love, nurturing, affirmation, and protection the child lacked as well as the present-day fulfillment (in work, relationships, and meaningful pastimes) that the adult requires. If you've let go of your painful emotions and have silenced the inner critic but are still not getting your adult and child needs met, you'll be compelled to continue overeating. Meeting the real needs of the child within is the third task of the four-pronged approach to healing addiction, and pursuing true fulfillment as an adult is the final task in this approach. (As you continue to read, there will be more on these tasks.)

Lenore's Story

I remember Lenore, a woman whose single mother had selfishly leaned on her and then finally abandoned her while she was still young. Lenore had never been taken care of so she grew up with very little understanding of how to care for herself. She was full of pain over her hard life.

She used starchy food as a way to soothe herself and to stuff down her hurt, anger, and sadness over having been exploited and abandoned. Lenore had been terrified to connect with her feelings, believing that she might "lose it" if she let herself access what was buried deep inside. Our work in therapy helped her find the strength to acknowledge her feelings and heal her wounds. After years of unsuccessful seesaw dieting, she was able to release her pain and feel confident enough to take care of herself. The need to use food as a comfort disappeared, followed by 60 pounds of excess weight.

It's not uncommon for someone to have at the same time a child within that's driving her to overeat and an internalized parent that makes her feel ashamed and guilty about this behavior. If this is you, I'm sure you've seen how the guilt and shame propel you right back to food for self-soothing. In order to stop overeating, your adult self has to reject the lies of the internalized parent and love and accept the child within right now. You must understand that you're not eating out of laziness or poor self-control but out of the child's misguided attempt at self-healing and self-nurturing. Doing this heals guilt and shame and breaks the vicious circle.

A child who doesn't receive adequate love, care, or protection from her parents or guardians will grow into an adult who's ambivalent about her unfulfilled needs. She'll be listening to the inner critic who tells her that she never really deserved to have her needs met or that her needs are excessive or shameful. These unmet needs are part of the child's emotional wounds. The child can't tolerate the pain of her unmet needs so she deals with it indirectly, pursuing illogical, ineffective solutions to what she needs. She'll go to these counterproductive solutions for two reasons: the first is that it's too confusing and frightening for the child within to face and pursue her needs directly. The second reason is that the child's simple nature is to go for the quick and easy answer, which usually happens to be a false one.

Each of these solutions for a child's real needs is what I call a "false fix," because they aren't valid means for the child within to obtain nurturing. Addictive behaviors are the only solutions she knows, however. Going after what she needs (even when unconscious and misguided) is a survival mechanism, which is why the child within can't let go of the false fixes.

Substitutes for the child's unmet emotional needs include food, alcohol, cigarettes, drugs, gambling, pornography, video games and compulsive spending. She associates these false fixes with healing and fulfillment because she's seen adults using them for this purpose. Observing your mother overeating, for example, made you unconsciously connect this activity with feeling better. Generation after generation observes its elders using these substitutes. This is one way addictions tend to run in families.

You might have also gotten the message from the media that one of these things could substitute for your unmet needs. You're a product of your family and your culture and if the media barrage you when you're young and impressionable with images of food being the next best thing to love, you'll internalize this message unconsciously.

Overeating is one of the most difficult addictions to deal with because you have to eat to survive and can always use this rationalization to continue overeating. A person who smokes, gambles, or takes drugs has no justification for these behaviors. You could completely give up most of the other substitutes and be better off, but you can't completely give up eating.

If you've unconsciously chosen food as a false fix, the issue is how to begin to see food not as the source of emotional fulfillment but as enjoyable nutrition. In order to do this, you'll need to find a constructive way to meet your emotional needs.

What makes a person unconsciously choose a particular love substitute or false fix? Why drink instead of gamble? Why overeat instead of using drugs? It could be because of parental or societal modeling. Sometimes, though, it's just something in your personality. For example, if you're very shy, you might choose drinking because it helps you feel more comfortable in social situations. If you have a competitive streak or feel hard done by, you might go for gambling to feel more powerful and in control. If you overeat compulsively, you could be hurt, angry, bored, lonely, or insecure and use food for soothing, stimulation, or distraction from unwanted emotions.

Since eating is a person's first and most powerful experience of feeling safe, soothed, and fulfilled, it tends to be a popular solution. The difference is usually in the degree to which a person uses it to meet her emotional needs and heal her wounds. Individuals with minor wounds might overindulge on occasion, while someone with a serious emotional wound might binge daily. Someone minimally wounded might use only one false fix occasionally, whereas someone significantly wounded might overeat, drink excessively, and overspend on a regular basis.

The choice of addiction can relate to your particular unmet needs: unconsciously, you'll seek out the solution that best seems to compensate for what you're missing. For example, if deep down, you need comfort and soothing, perhaps you'll turn to "comfort food"; if you need to numb your pain, maybe you'll take drugs; if you feel empty, you might try shopping to fill yourself up; if you feel needy, you might become addicted to relationships; and if you're anxious and need to calm your fears, you could turn to alcohol.

As I mentioned before, many people use more than one false fix, in part because addictions are interchangeable. Also, because none of these solutions give you what you need and all of them serve the same purpose, a person can go from one to another, forever trying and failing to meet her needs and heal her wounds.

Helping the child within face and grieve the losses she's experienced will help her to let go of her wounds. Giving her love and affirmation will stop the vicious circle the child perpetuates by avoiding her needs and feelings and then pursuing false solutions. The more you practice loving and healing the child within, the stronger you'll become as an adult and the more power you'll have to care for the child within and heal even her deepest wounds.

Still, because pain is involved, it won't be easy to face your wounds. From a child's perspective, needs and feelings are overwhelming and possibly dangerous to face, let alone express. For this reason, some people find that healing their wounds can be facilitated by working with well-trained, experienced professional counselors or therapists. These individuals can help you feel safe enough to connect to your unconscious material and can help you learn how to replace the false fixes with real solutions.

We talked about the wounds that come from unmet needs, which come from the *lack* of love, care, or protection needed in childhood, but there are also wounds that come from the *presence* of something negative when you were growing up. I call these "wounding experiences."

We're extremely sensitive to our childhood experiences. Our young brains are still developing, and the brain is an organ that changes in response to its environment. This will happen in the same way that growing bones will become misshapen if there's a lack of vitamin D during childhood or that developing teeth will be permanently stained if a child is given certain antibiotics to treat an infection.

If you've lived through abuse, rejection, exploitation, or humiliation, then you'll have developed emotional wounds. As I mentioned previously, a wound can manifest as low self-esteem, poor self-confidence, or difficulties with work or relationships. It can also appear as the fear of abandonment, a need for control, severe self-criticism, or the expectation of failure. It can come out as cynicism, irritability, pessimism, or feeling lonely even when others are around. You can see it in the experience of passivity, indecisiveness, self-centeredness, and general malaise.

If you've experienced any wounding experiences in your childhood, they were made worse because there was nothing you could have done to change things. In fact, the only thing you would have had to hold on to was the hope that things could change.

If a child feels powerless to change the people or situations around her, she can lose all hope and her suffering can become unbearable. Her only hope is in trying to *change herself.* This gives her the will to go on because she can hold onto the hope that if she were a better child, she'd be treated differently by her caregivers.

The act of hoping was the way a child might survive a situation in which she felt otherwise utterly hopeless and helpless. Hoping to change and thereby have others respond to her differently became a powerful survival tool and took a prominent place in the child's mind. Even though it was never fulfilled, the child's hope gave her a reason to live and that's why she can't let it go. This primitive survival tool becomes the pathological hope of the child within.

When you're an adult, pathological hope is an exercise in futility. You now have the power to change situations or walk away from hurtful people. Still, until you become conscious of this false hope, the child within is compelled to cling to it. If you're a compulsive eater, the hope could be demonstrated by the child within seeing the next binge or the one after it as that which will finally heal her. You're going to have to replace the hope with a solution that actually works.

Eating is complicated because it's the very first thing you took in after your first breath. You've used it since birth to soothe yourself, fill yourself, calm your fears, and connect you to your mother—your original source of love. It is the most primitive activity a person can engage in and one of the most deeply satisfying. Eating is an experience that's charged with an enormous amount of meaning and memories.

It's easy for the child within to turn to compulsive eating because food is seen as the original cure-all. You eat something and feel better for a while and the child within hopes that more food will fix her wounds and fulfill her needs once and for all.

The child within drives you to overeat and for a moment, you feel satisfied. Your experience of fullness reminds you of nursing as an infant in your mother's arms, and brings back feelings you may never have felt since. If you keep on eating, though, the initially pleasant sensation becomes an experience of overfullness, often accompanied by critical messages from the internalized parent. Your moment of peace, pleasure, and satisfaction has been transformed into an experience of self-recrimination, remorse, and even self-punishment by the inner critic.

There's another important issue at play in the battle to lose weight and keep it off. Earlier in chapter 1 I mentioned Lucinda, a young woman who'd become extremely anxious when she'd begun losing weight. In the course of therapy, Lucinda realized that because of her history of abuse as a child, she had an unconscious terror of entering into relationships because she expected to be rejected. She didn't feel able to tolerate any more pain. She saw, through therapy, that she'd been using her weight to keep potential friends or romantic partners at bay. The problem was that her weight wasn't an effective deterrent to friends or men.

Lucinda was a lovely person and people wanted to get to know her, regardless of what she weighed. She started to make friends and to date, but then trouble arose because she'd been depending on her weight to protect her and hadn't learned how to take care of herself in her relationships. Lucinda didn't know how to choose the right kind of people to associate with or how to express her needs and feelings. She had a few bad experiences that made her want even more to hold onto the weight, believing that this symbolic "buffer zone" could keep her safe.

Through therapy, Lucinda learned that her weight was an ineffective defense against being hurt and she began, instead, to develop the adult empowerment and self-trust that would enable her to feel safe in her relationships. Once she felt secure in this way, Lucinda no longer "needed" the extra weight, because she was replacing a defective protection with effective tools for dealing with people.

Lucinda was *psychologically attached to her weight,* and many people share this defense. In such individuals, the frightened child within believes that she needs to hide behind the symbolic wall of the weight. For someone who was abused or exploited as a child and desperately fears further suffering, being very large may, paradoxically, make her less visible in a society that notices what it idealizes and ignores the less-than-ideal.

Some people use the extra weight as an excuse for failures in their work life or in intimate relationships. As I mentioned before, if you've grown up being made to feel that you're unlovable, you may come to expect rejection. The child within is convinced that she can blame the fat for any rejection she might encounter. This way, at least she had control over *why* she was rejected. She can say, "they hate the fat, not me."

If a child grows up being made to feel that she isn't intelligent or competent, the child within can think, "I can't do this is because I'm fat," or, "I failed at this because of my weight, and not because I'm inadequate." The child within alleviates her intolerable anxiety over potential rejection or failure by manufacturing an excuse for it in advance.

THE STORY OF BESS

Bess was a researcher who'd had the horrible experience of being molested as a child. She grew up unconsciously believing that she'd been victimized because she was too pretty or sexy. Children personalize what happens to them and the child within Bess was convinced that she was *guilty* of inciting the abuse.

Some women become large to neutralize their attractiveness or sexuality. As an adult, Bess gained weight so that she'd no longer stir up lust in men that she was convinced they couldn't control. The child within her believed that being big would make her less vulnerable around men and safer in her body and in the world. Unfortunately, as with all child-driven coping strategies, gaining weight didn't make Bess feel any safer. It was only through our work in therapy that she was able to develop trust in her own ability to take care of herself and feel confident, empowered, and *innocent* around men. It was at that point that the weight began to fall off.

Often, a woman will become overweight because of obvious or subtle pressure from family members, friends, or romantic partners. These individuals consciously or unconsciously want her to be heavy. A parent may prefer you to be overweight because they want to continue to baby you and keep you dependent on them. Sometimes a sister or a friend is threatened by what she sees as sexual competition and would rather you weren't thin and desirable to men.

A romantic partner might be afraid that if you were thinner, other men would find you attractive and you'd be tempted to stray. This type of partner might believe that if you were more confident in your body, you'd have no reason to not act on this temptation. In this person's mind, your extra weight is insurance against infidelity.

All these people profess to love and care about you but they're sabotaging your attempts to break free of your eating and weight problems. You need to see them as the "outer opponents" they are, and no longer allow them to undermine your attempts to let go of the extra weight. Of course, in order to do this, you have to stop colluding with anyone who's invested in your remaining overweight.

You need to see that staying heavy to make others happy is a lose–lose proposition. It won't give them what they really need—which is to deal with their competitiveness, jealousy, or insecurity, and trying to please others by remaining fat won't heal your wounds, either. Whether your need to be heavy is coming from the inside or outside, you have to become conscious of it to let it go.

Whatever meaning or purpose that the weight has for you, you'll have to find a better way to provide yourself with this. If not, you might temporarily become thinner but the weight will always come back, because it's *needed*. You need to see that if you're significantly overweight, there are really two problems you have to work on when you're trying to resolve your issues with eating and weight: the need to overeat compulsively and the need to carry the extra weight. Both must be fully resolved if you're to lose weight and keep it off permanently.

VISUALIZATION 1: DEVELOPING THE ADULT IDENTITY (MEETING THE CHILD WITHIN)

One tool that's extremely helpful in enabling you to develop your adult identity is a visualization exercise that allows you to connect to the child within. When you use your active imagination to meet the child within and establish a relationship with her, you'll simultaneously be growing the adult identity, because it's the adult part that interacts with the child. The more you practice connecting with the child within, the more you'll be strengthening your adult identity at the same time.

Begin the visualization by first making yourself comfortable in a straight-backed chair. Remove your shoes, watch, and eyeglasses so that you can focus inward, and feel your feet on the ground. Focus your attention on your breathing and let your breaths be slow and deep. Now, picture yourself seated in a beautiful, comfortable armchair, in a small, cozy room. The chair is the most beautiful, comfortable one you could possibly imagine.

Notice that directly across from where you're sitting is a small, low door and that up and to the right of this door is a full-length mirror with a beautiful, ornate gilded frame. To the left of the small door and high on the wall is a small round window, and directly under this window, standing on the floor against the wall are three tall earthenware urns. Otherwise, the room is bare.

Bring your attention now to the small door. Notice that it's beginning to open. You see a small figure coming into the room. It's the child within. Notice how old she is and her appearance. Is she walking or crawling, entering the room enthusiastically or reluctantly? Does she have a smile on her face or a sad or angry look? Pay attention to what you're feeling as you encounter this child part of you. Are you happy, nervous, excited? Ask the child to come to you and to sit with you in the beautiful, comfortable chair.

Notice if the child is willing or not to approach you; does she come right up and sit with you in the chair, or does she come only partway and stand there, looking up at you? Allow her to do what's right for her. You are, after all, just meeting for the first time. Take a moment to feel what it's like to see the child within right in front of you, and to observe her reaction to you. Sometimes this child will be angry toward the adult self, and that's because she feels abandoned by you.

You've haven't done anything wrong; it's just that you weren't aware of her existence and therefore haven't been in contact with her until now. If the child appears upset at you, acknowledge her feelings and promise her that you'll never leave her again. Tell the child that now that you've met, you'll always be there for her. Pay attention to how this makes her feel. See if this enables her to approach you more closely.

Now, tell the child how happy you are to finally meet her, and ask if there's anything she wants from you right now. Listen very closely to what she says, and do your best to respond with love and compassion. She might not trust you yet and she might need a lot of reassurance that you won't abandon her again. (You'll probably have to do this exercise a number of times, until the child within feels perfectly safe with you.) If she's sitting with you, cuddle with the child and let her see that you really care. Tell her that you're going to do everything from now on to be take care of her and give her the nurturing and healing that she needs.

If the child isn't sitting with you, now let her go back through the small door. If she's on the chair with you, hold her close and bring her right up against your heart. Notice that she's beginning to shimmer and glimmer and become transparent. Press her to your chest, and feel the child entering your heart. Her beautiful child energy is filling your heart with love. Feel what it's like to have the child within residing in your heart, knowing that you want only the best for this beautiful creature and that you'll always be connected to her.

Now it's time to come back to reality. Feel the child in your heart, or if she left through the small door, feel the trace of her presence and know that you'll meet her again soon. Know that eventually, she'll trust you enough to come up on the chair with you, sit in your lap and enter your heart. Take a moment with your feelings, having met the child within, and notice if you're crying. This is a normal response and a healing one so let the tears flow. When you're ready, open your eyes and return to reality. Know that you can revisit this small, cozy room whenever you want, and can spend time here with the child within whenever you choose.

4

The Road to Healing: Obstacles, Wrong Turns, and Finding Your Way

The 12 Miss-Steps

My patient Lulu, a lawyer who's been struggling with overeating for many years, told me a story about her experience with the 12 Steps. She'd been part of a group of about a dozen women, all trying to lose weight at Overeaters Anonymous (OA). Out of the entire group, only one woman, Jerry, had lost weight, and this woman ended up becoming a compulsive calorie counter and food restrictor, substituting compulsively controlled eating for compulsive overeating. Of all the women in her OA group, Jerry, who'd been "successful" at losing weight, was the unhappiest member and seemed to be even more obsessive in her thinking about food and weight than when she was heavy. Lulu quit the group in despair and began therapy with me.

Because of stories like these, I have a philosophical problem with the 12 Step program. It's based on concepts that in this day and age no longer seem relevant. Most importantly, it views every addict as being helpless in the face of their problem, with healing only possible through giving up one's power to an external "higher being." This is contrary to my view that addiction is the problem of someone who isn't empowered, and for whom reclaiming their power is the key to letting go of addiction.

The 12 Step philosophy errs, in my mind, in that it groups together members on the basis of their failings. I think that focusing on your failings is counterproductive in the healing of addiction because it promotes helplessness and shame—two of the main forces driving addiction, in my opinion.

As I said previously, I disagree with the disease model of addiction. I see addiction not as a disease but as a misguided solution with regard to emotional needs and healing. A disease is something that happens to you beyond your control, whereas addiction is something that you've chosen to do—albeit unconsciously—and can consciously choose to let go of. The model of personal helplessness in addiction is what, I believe, perpetuates the addictive behavior, whereas a philosophy of personal responsibility makes it possible for an addict to be empowered around overcoming their addiction.

It seems evident that the disease model was adopted in order to decrease the stigma on addicts by seeing them not as "bad," "lazy," or "self-indulgent," but as people who are "afflicted" with their addiction. This model is unnecessary if we can simply have compassion for the wounded child within each addict who is desperately trying to heal her traumatic or deficient past through the misguided solution of addiction.

According to the 12 Step philosophy, your addiction is a chronic disease that you'll have to spend your entire life fighting "one day at a time," but that's okay, because they'll give you the support to keep on fighting it. This runs counter to my experience in which people have been able to fully let go of addiction without it being a daily struggle when they've dealt with the unfinished business of their past. Proponents of the 12 Step philosophy have convinced their adherents that they're helpless in the face of addiction, where no one can ever really graduate from the program and get on with their life, but are doomed forever to be an "addict," who must always belong to the organization.

The disease model says that every addict is a victim of her problem and that the problem is greater than she is. Well, this is true on one level: *the addiction is more powerful than the child within.* This child does need a stronger force to help her overcome addiction. Where my thinking differs from the disease model is in the knowledge and experience that each person has an adult identity that they can step into through their healing work, and that *the adult self is far more powerful than any addiction.*

This adult identity has all the strength the child within needs for you to overcome any addiction. You won't forever have to fight the obsessive thoughts and compulsive urges associated with addiction. Healing your wounds and becoming an empowered adult will make addiction unnecessary because you'll have found real, meaningful ways to nurture yourself and be happy. By doing the work of healing, there will be no need to struggle forever against the addiction, and rather than perpetually being "in recovery," you can finally be fully recovered.

I see many flaws in the disease model and in the way people are counseled that they can't leave the program and stay sober. In a sense, the 12 Step program is similar to a cult, where the members are passive recipients of the great and mighty wisdom of the leaders and must give up their personal power and submit to the will of a "higher power" or to those in charge. The members can never leave and must spend their lives serving the organization.

Members of 12 Step programs sometimes even disconnect from their loved ones if these people don't support what they're doing, and at the same time they try to bring their friends and family into the organization to be in offshoots of it, like Al-Anon.

The 12 Step programs say that addicts who relapse are "not following the program." In fact, it seems much more likely that it's the program that has failed the addicts who need a much better form of treatment in order to be free of their addiction.

It's impossible to find reliable statistics on the success of 12 Step based rehab programs. A best, it appears that perhaps only 3–5 percent of people who go through these programs actually stay recovered in the long run, and in the short term, the dropout rate is enormous. Of those who stay in rehab, few become sober, many relapse, and many people credit the 12 Step program for their sobriety when in fact it had nothing to do with it.

These people mistakenly believe that their recovery is due to their participation in Alcoholics Anonymous (AA), Narcotics Anonymous (NA), or OA, but often they're wrong. What I believe really happened is that they were doing some meaningful healing work at the same time as they attended a 12 Step program, and it was this work that enabled them to let go of their addiction. *If you're in a 12 Step program at the same time as you become able to let go of your addiction, it doesn't mean that this is what's responsible for your success.*

Many people are simultaneously in a 12 Step program and some other sort of therapy and I credit the therapy for their recovery. The 12 Step program gets the credit, however, because it's specifically focused on helping people let go of *addiction.* Any psychotherapy, counseling, or coaching these people might be doing won't be credited for their recovery but, in fact, it's healing their emotional wounds and learning real self-soothing and self-nurturing that will allow a person to break free from her addictions, as opposed to any 12 Step program.

It's interesting to note that there is no way to really assess the effectiveness of this type of treatment for addiction. AA keeps its own statistics but we have to take them with a grain of salt. Many of us have witnessed a friend or family member going through the revolving door of rehab, only to return again and again after each failure to maintain sobriety. It's so unfortunate that a program with such a poor track record would be considered the gold standard for dealing with addiction. It also saddens me that the individuals going through the program without the benefit of real, effective therapy would be blamed for failing at the 12 Steps, rather than anyone looking at what's wrong with these steps. Most unfortunate is the fact that this type of program has become such a sacred cow that it's very controversial to question it. That's too bad because it needs to be questioned or people will continue to use it with the same dismal results.

One good thing about organizations such as AA, NA, or OA is that they provide addicts with community. However, the bad things about belonging to this community are many. For example, if your sponsor falls off the wagon, which is not uncommon, it's frightening and demoralizing and could make you believe that it's more difficult than you thought to stay sober. If the group says that you must come to meetings forever in order to stay sober, then you can never leave the group. You must spend the rest of your life identified as "an addict," rather than a free and empowered person who's pursuing positive goals.

I've seen too many people go through months and even years of so-called rehabilitation, both as inpatients and on the outside in 12 Step programs, only to fall back into addiction. The program has failed them because it misses the fundamental point in dealing with addiction: that an addict is driven to the compulsive behavior and obsessive thinking around their false solution of addiction by the deep wounds they incurred in childhood. If these wounds aren't acknowledged and addressed, how is an addict ever to break free of the problem?

The 12 Step philosophy has the wrong goal: sobriety. In AA, for example, the goal is to get you to give up drinking completely. What isn't stressed is having the alcoholic look at what deeper needs and wounds are driving them to drink, what the drinking means to them, or for what it might be compensating. Without understanding the meaning and purpose of the alcohol addiction and without providing the tools for psychological healing and nurturing that replace the misguided choice of drinking, there's no way that the alcoholic will be able to quit. The 12 Step philosophy values the use of *willpower* in achieving sobriety, whereas I value the *power of healing the wounds* driving addiction.

The 12 Step program encourages the addict to surrender to a higher power to find sobriety. I see this as the opposite of healing. If you're truly to heal the wounds underlying your addictive behavior, the adult self must become strong and take its rightful place at the forefront of your personality, and as I said previously, learn to face, grieve, and let go of the wounds that are driving your compulsive behavior and find real, valid ways to love and nurture the child within and to pursue adult fulfillment.

Joining the 12 Step movement is essentially trading one master for another. The first master, the cruel and critical internalized parent is replaced by the second master, the "higher power" to whom each member must surrender her will. There's little room in this philosophy for the empowerment of the individual or for real healing of the deepest layers of addiction. Even if by joining this movement you could give up one addiction, you'd only end up replacing it with another one because the wounds driving your compulsive behavior and obsessive thinking haven't been dealt with. It makes a person feel that much more overwhelmed by the enormity of the problem when she's told that she's powerless in the face of her problem. You aren't powerless unless you *choose* to give up your adult power.

In fact, it may not be necessary to completely give up drinking if you were truly healed of your addiction. Healing means freedom from the obsessive thinking about drinking and from the compulsive need to drink excessively. If you've let go of the wounds of the past and have learned how to give yourself the love and care you truly need, I can see you being able to drink in moderation. In fact, I have patients who do so. Overeaters can't give up food completely and yet they're expected, by working the OA program, to learn to eat in moderation.

In fact, my patient Megan, who is 14 years sober from a very severe narcotics addiction, recently was in a bad car accident and incurred some serious injuries. In the emergency department, she was given Demerol, a narcotic painkiller. This was the first time she'd used anything stronger than an aspirin or acetaminophen since she's been sober. At first, she refused the medication, terrified that this would be the beginning of a downward spiral into relapse, but then she had an epiphany: she remembered that she'd always used drugs to numb her pain, and that the therapy she's been doing has enabled her to create a great life for herself. She realized that she was happy and fulfilled, and that she had no urge whatsoever to take up drugs again.

I imagine that the 12 Step people had a problem with the concept of moderation. The "temptation" is always there with food, whereas AA, NA, or Gamblers Anonymous (GA) members are told to abstain completely from their addiction of choice and avoid "temptation." If you look at the statistics, however, OA members are no less successful than the other groups, even when faced with temptation on a daily basis.

If food is your addictive substance of choice, needing to eat every day doesn't make you any more likely to fail in letting go of the addiction than a drinker who could completely avoid temptation. Overcoming addiction lies in healing emotional wounds and not in trying to avoid the problem substance or activity. Unless the substance or activity is dangerous, illegal, or causes physical dependency, I believe that healing from an addiction can ultimately allow someone to have a normal relationship with the subject of their addiction. Alcoholics can heal enough to have an occasional social drink, shopaholics can enter a store without spraining their credit cards, and overeaters can eat normally, without having to exert enormous willpower every time they're around food.

It's true that there's a physiological component to alcohol abuse, but that's resolved through physical detoxification. What remains is the craving that comes from the emotional wound. When this issue is resolved, an alcoholic can theoretically have a normal relationship with alcohol. In the same way, a food addict can learn to have a normal relationship with food.

Some diet plans say that this is impossible, and that you'll forever be restricting portions, counting calories, and eating "boring food" to avoid the temptation to overindulge. What a miserable life that would be. Depriving yourself of the pleasure of eating is an unnecessary sacrifice. Why give up your power to a 12 Step program, or any type of diet, when you can achieve real freedom by finally dealing with your emotional needs and wounds. In this way, a former overeater can find pleasure in good food without being in a dysfunctional relationship with it, and an alcoholic can learn to enjoy a glass of wine without needing to finish the bottle.

More often than not, someone going through a 12 Step program will experience the *transfer of addictions.* A drinker becomes a smoker, an overeater becomes a shopper, or a cocaine addict becomes a gambler. As I mentioned previously, it's easy to go from one dysfunctional coping mechanism to another as the child within becomes extremely anxious when she's deprived of her only source of healing and nurturing and is desperate to replace it with something else.

The only way to avoid this transference of addictions is to heal the wounds at the heart of the addiction, as opposed to being perpetually "in recovery."

The goal is to be free of all compulsive behavior and obsessive thinking around addiction. Lulu's acquaintance, Jerry, who lost all her weight while in OA, was still compulsive in her food restriction and still obsessed with food and weight. She was locked in the prison of addiction and even more unhappy than she had been while heavy. In my mind that has nothing to do with healing.

Healing of addiction ought to take place in an atmosphere of loving kindness and ruthless honesty. Each individual must be seen as responsible for the consequences of her actions and choices, but doesn't require the punishment of an internal or external parent-figure for these choices. No outside power is needed to impose sobriety on a person, or to take away his or her supposed "defects," as one of the 12 Steps refers to.

Here's a different method for dealing with addiction. It lays out 10 basic truths that will enable you to achieve freedom from any addiction. For those who overeat, I believe that it's the ideal method for achieving lasting change. You could replace the 12 Steps with these 10 truths:

First Truth: I realize that I'm an adult who is responsible for her choices and for the consequences of these choices.

Second Truth: I recognize that some of the choices I've made have hurt me and others, and I need to make better choices.

Third Truth: I acknowledge that these hurtful choices have come from wounds deep within me, and that in order to make better choices, I must address these wounds.

Fourth Truth: I admit to myself that my emotional wounds come from losses I experienced during childhood: of love, validation, protection, and innocence, and that I must deal with these losses to heal my wounds.

Fifth Truth: I accept that addiction is a dysfunctional way of dealing with past losses, and that no matter how much I engage in it, my wounds can't be healed in this way.

Sixth Truth: I understand that true healing from addiction involves letting go of both my obsessive thinking about this false solution and my compulsion to engage in it.

Seventh Truth: I trust that I have the strength and courage to face the losses of my childhood, to grieve them, and let them go in order to move through the healing process.

Eighth Truth: I know that I'm the only person who can compensate for my childhood losses, and I promise to be there for myself in this way.

Ninth Truth: I see that healing my wounds, providing myself with the love and care I was deprived of in childhood, and becoming free of obsessive thinking and compulsive behavior are what will enable me to make better choices in the future.

Tenth Truth: I see that letting go of addiction includes choosing to focus on discovering and pursuing my true dreams and on being a positive, contributing member of my community.

Addiction to Dieting (How Dieting Is a False Solution, Engaged in Compulsively)

My patient Lucinda lost 100 pounds on an extremely restricted-calorie diet. Her body changed a lot and she began getting attention from men. At this point she panicked, quit the program, and despite all the money she spent to lose the weight, she promptly gained back the 100 pounds, plus interest.

The diet doctor Lucinda had consulted never sat down and talked to her about what the extra weight meant for her, or what feelings were coming up when she began to lose the weight. This doctor never learned about Lucinda's powerful psychological attachment to the extra weight and her need to protect herself against feeling vulnerable in relationships.

Without having this crucial piece of information about Lucinda and without being able to provide her with other, more effective tools for feel safer in her personal interactions, any diet plan was doomed to fail. It was only in therapy that Lucinda was able to stop berating herself for having "wasted" her money on this "sure-fire" diet program and to see that she first had to address her fears of being thinner before she could let go of her extra weight.

According to Lucinda, the diet doctor applied the same weight-loss "plan" to each person who came to the program, regardless of what was going on in her psyche, as though every overweight person had exactly the same reasons for being heavy, which was that they ate too much. Both the program this doctor was providing and, really, all other diets on the market today are just businesses out to make a profit. The diet industry makes promises that your needs will be met if you follow its plan, but it can't live up to these promises.

There's a lot of money to be made in the diet business and these programs are competing with each other for it. Each program tells you, "I'll fix you. I'll change your life for the better. It's quick and easy my way." The language of these programs plays right in to the child's pathological hope and her need for instant, easy results.

They also echo the internalized parent's demands that you lose your "shameful" and "unsightly" weight. The child within, if she's eager to please the parent, will at first pursue her diet as compulsively as she pursues her overeating. Eventually, though, the deprivation, frustration, and self-criticism involved in dieting will result in a failure to lose weight or to keep off any weight that had been lost.

When the child within is in charge of your love life, you become prey for the charming con artist who promises to rescue you and then instead controls and oppresses you for his own unscrupulous purposes. In the same way, if the adult isn't in charge of your relationship to food and weight, you'll be vulnerable to the diet programs that promise you that you can lose weight without expending any real effort.

Effort isn't something a child wants to expend, except on making sure she has a rescuer or some sort of quick fix handy. The child within is seduced by the false promises of charismatic charmers or well-publicized diet programs, believing that these will bring her the healing and happiness she needs. Abusive lovers promise to take care of you but in the end, you're exploited and abandoned. Diet programs promise to rescue you from the prison of your extra weight but abuse your trust, take your money, and abandon you emotionally. Both promise to give you what you want but neither will give you what you need.

Every diet plan is alike in that it promises you that it alone will fix your problem. You're told that you can't lose weight without doing this particular diet. Each program tells you exactly what, when, and how to eat. It controls everything you put in your mouth and blames, shames, and criticizes you if you don't do exactly what the rules say. You're made to feel "weak," "lazy," "lacking in willpower," or "undisciplined" if you can't comply. It insists that it's always your fault if you fail at a diet and never the fault of the diet itself. Have you ever once seen a diet program take responsibility for its failure in meeting your needs?

If you believe in the diet and try to follow its rules, it's like being with a bad lover: you'll abdicate adult responsibility for yourself and give your power to the diet plan. You hope that it will cure your overeating and enable you to lose weight, but you can never be "good enough." When the diet eventually fails, and they all do, you'll feel bad about yourself. You'll either give up in despair or try again, either with the same diet or with another plan, with the same compulsiveness with which you pursued overeating. It's easy to become as *addicted to dieting* as you've been to food, but no matter how many times you try to make a diet work, it won't, because diets are not the way to overcome compulsive eating or to let go of extra weight.

These programs might make you feel like a failure, but in reality each diet has failed you. Like many who diet, you might have become frustrated with yourself and more and more hopeless about your ability to lose weight. Your self-esteem sinks every time you fail at a diet or every time you regain the weight that you'd previously lost. You've probably gone from one diet to another in the pathological hope that dieting could enable you finally to lose the weight and keep it off. Like so many, you believed the false promises of the diet programs because you desperately wanted the answer to be "out there." It's not your fault. Nobody told you the truth: the answer was always within you.

You didn't know that the reason you can't lose the weight is because diets don't give you the tools you need to create lasting change. No diet plan can help you understand and heal the wounds that are driving the compulsive eating and the weight gain or discover the things in life that bring real fulfillment. Until you stop believing in the false promises of these diets, you won't be able to see that your post-diet weight gain is due to the child within sabotaging your efforts because she's angry about being deprived or in despair of ever meeting an impossible goal. Dieting only reinforces the child's need for real healing, love, and fulfillment.

The diet industry capitalizes on the desperation and denial of those individuals whose child is in charge and exploits exactly the same compulsiveness that the child brings to her overeating. You're enticed into one diet after another. Every month or so, a new book is published on how to lose weight the quick and easy way. Several times a week, there's an ad or story on TV or the Internet promoting the latest diet "secrets." It's clear from this that not one of these diets actually works because, as I said previously, if any one did, there'd be no market for the next one, and the one after that. Still, in our pathological hope and refusal to see the lies being promulgated, too many of us are still buying up all the books, following every new diet, and inevitably failing.

My patient Eloise was taken on by a "diet doctor" when she was a teenager standing 5 feet, 5 inches tall and weighing 135 pounds. She was put on a 600-calorie-a-day diet and told that this was going to help her. According to her family doctor, the average weight for her height was 138 pounds, which means that she was low-to-normal in weight. Even so, this diet doctor took a still-growing girl into the program and severely restricted her caloric intake for several weeks. As a result, her metabolism was almost permanently damaged, and it's only been in middle age that she's been able, finally, to get her metabolism and weight back to normal.

You will no longer be at risk of being the victim of unscrupulous diet programs if you choose to wake up and to grow up; to let go of your desperation and denial and take responsibility for your own healing. Giving up your adult power and allowing others to have control over your diet (or your love life, for that matter) makes you helpless and perpetuates your unhappiness and anger, encouraging addiction. Taking charge of your life, dealing with your wounds, and pursuing your adult dreams will enable you to be free from addiction and free from exploitation, whether from diet programs or charming, destructive lovers.

Gina's Story

A patient of mine named Gina, a lovely nurse with a severe overeating problem, used to take pride in how nice and helpful she was to others. Unfortunately, people kept taking advantage of her generosity and frequently treated her with disrespect. Gina didn't understand why this was happening, so she tried even harder to be nice in the hope that the people around her would eventually reciprocate. All the while, Gina was putting on more and more weight.

So many women, just like Gina, have been taught to believe that being "nice" is the right way to be. They were taught to please others and placate conflict or learned to behave in these ways as a survival mechanism in the face of neglect or abuse.

Women are frequently overly invested in being likable and avoiding confrontation. In a loving family environment, the child grows up to develop confidence and feels secure in the knowledge that she's acceptable just as she is. In an emotionally deprived environment, the child grows up feeling unlovable, because it's her nature to believe that she's the cause of whatever's happening to her. She blames herself for what are, in fact, the shortcomings of her parents or guardians. She reasons, in her child-logic, that if she were only a better, nicer, more helpful child, then surely things would be different.

Unfortunately, when this unloved child grows into an adult, the child within persists in believing that if she were nicer or better, then she'd be loved and healed. In her child heart, she hopes that if she pleases the people in her life today, the love she receives will make up for what she didn't get while growing up. If the child grew up around abuse, she'll have learned to placate the anger of her parent(s) to stay safe. She'll have gotten very good at this and will grow up convinced that she still needs this survival mechanism as an adult. She believes that placating others' anger and avoiding confrontation will prevent people from withdrawing from her or hurting her.

If this is you, you need to see that pleasing the people in your life today will never heal the wounds of the child within. No matter how they feel toward you, it'll have no effect on the child. Love that was lost in the past can't be compensated for with love today, and healing can only happen when you grieve your losses, put the past behind you, and learn to love and care for yourself. The "nice" child will never get what she's looking for by pleasing others and she'll remain emotionally hungry. The child within will be driven to overeat in order to feed this persistent hunger for love.

Pleasing and placating others will often cause them to treat you in exactly the opposite way you hoped for. People are sensitive to the weakness of others, and some individuals see pleasing or placating behavior as evidence that you're weak or needy. These people will take advantage of your vulnerability. At best they'll disrespect you and at worst, they'll attempt to exploit or abuse you. Rather than ingratiating yourself with the people in your life, you'll often end up being mistreated by them. This will cause you to feel hurt and angry and if you have a tendency to turn to food for soothing, it'll make you hungry.

Some people see those who please and placate as emotionally threatening. These individuals are uncomfortable with their own vulnerability or neediness and when you demonstrate the need to please, they see their own needy child within reflected in your behavior. You're inadvertently mirroring to them a side of themselves that they can't tolerate seeing, so they'll be hostile toward you as a defense against the disowned fragility that you're bringing to their attention. The more you try to please them, the more likely they are to be abusive toward you.

In cases of pleasing and placating, the adult part of the psyche has to let the child part know that being nice and avoiding confrontation will not win her love or prevent her from being hurt. In fact, a pleaser is just the kind of person a manipulative user is looking for and very often, pleasers attract exploitative, uncaring people into their lives.

Gina didn't realize that she was setting herself up to be disrespected by people because of her overly nice behavior. She didn't see, until she came to therapy, that the result of trying to please others is to end up feeling more used than loved. When you're busy being nice, you're not only missing out on the love you need but you're also agreeing to things you'd rather not do. You're wasting a lot of energy trying to please, and constantly wondering whether people like you or if you've inadvertently done something to upset them.

All of this will ultimately cause the child within to become resentful. In typical child-logic, the same child who wants so badly to please others gets angry at having to go along with what everyone else wants. The child within really doesn't like having to take the "emotional temperature" of everyone around her. It's a huge burden for the child to be constantly checking on how the other people in her life are reacting to her, and then adjusting her behavior accordingly.

This resentment is for the most part unconscious because the need to be loved is so great that the child couldn't tolerate facing the anger that's building up inside her. If she faced her anger it might cause her to stop being nice, and that just wouldn't do for the child who sees pleasing as the only way she can finally be loved. If you're a pleaser, it's likely that your unconscious resentment will build and build and eventually, your resentment will leak out in passive-aggressive behavior, or you'll have to stuff it down with food.

Passive-aggressive behavior is anger expressed indirectly. This happens when a person can't face her own anger or is afraid of making others angry if she shows her true feelings. The anger becomes locked in the unconscious, so she's not aware when she's "leaking."

For example, a person being passive-aggressive will arrive late for an appointment, "accidentally" break the dish she's washing, or neglect the houseplants. He might forget to pay a bill or borrow and lose your favorite scarf. These people believe that they didn't mean to do harm, but deep down inside, they did, as they needed to vent their anger. When a woman is trying to be "nice" but is also leaking resentment in passive-aggressive behavior, her mixed messages will confuse the people around her. If they weren't hostile with her to begin with, her passive-aggressive behavior will make them angry.

This will cause the woman great distress, as her aim was the opposite: to avoid confrontation and obtain affection. Because she's unconscious of the resentment brewing inside of her, she won't be able to stop being passive-aggressive. If she keeps making the people in her life angry, she could easily turn to overeating as a way of comforting and soothing herself.

Pleasing and placating don't work. The only way to know if others like you is by being yourself. It's only by being genuine that you can trust that the people around you truly care for you. If you're a pleaser, all you can know is that others might enjoy or appreciate what you do for them, but you'll have no way of knowing if they care. The same goes for avoiding confrontation.

Gina told me a story about a friend of hers named Lara. Lara wanted to go to an upcoming singles' dance and was pressuring Gina to go with her, but Gina didn't want to go. Gina told me that she was considering giving in to her friend's wishes and going to the dance anyway, because she was "afraid of the consequences" if she didn't.

This is what I told her: "A real friend can tolerate it when you say 'No.' The way you can tell a real friend from a user is by saying 'No' when you need to. Real friends don't need you to go along with everything they want; they just need you to care about them, take an interest in them, and get along with them. Anyone who gets angry at you when you say 'No,' is showing you that they're a false friend."

Gina decided to tell her friend that she wouldn't be going to the dance, and it turns out that her friend was fine with it. Gina's fear of repercussions had to do with her assumption that Lara was as demanding and unreasonable as Gina's parents had always been. In reality, Lara was a caring and reasonable friend.

Lisa's Story

Recently, I've been working with an actress named Lisa who was abruptly left by her partner of several years. Lisa was shocked at his sudden, inexplicable departure. But in retrospect, it's clear what happened: she had gotten involved in a type of relationship that's doomed from the start. Lisa had been a pleaser and had a partner who was a user.

The problem with this type of relationship is that both the pleaser and user are being driven by the needs of the child within. The child within the pleaser is trying to heal her wounds by getting the person she pleases to love her, and the child within the user is trying to get his wounds healed by getting the other person to please him.

This codependent type of relationship can't work, not only because the pleaser will never be loved for all her caretaking, but because the user, no matter how much he receives, will *never be satisfied* with what the pleaser is offering. Just as the pleaser can't heal her wounds of childhood by getting someone to love her today, the user can't compensate for the love he didn't receive as a child by exploiting another person. The child within each of them needs to be loved by the adult self. It's the responsibility of every adult to deal with their persistent emotional wounds and needs.

After years of being in relationship with Lisa, her partner got tired of unsuccessfully trying to get his needs met. He blamed her and called her useless, making her feel like a failure. Lisa had believed that her niceness would be met with love but ultimately, it was met with rejection. She was left feeling that she was to blame for the relationship ending.

Lisa's partner had telephoned her after he left, saying that if only she'd been able to give him what he needed, he wouldn't have had to leave. He might believe this but it's not true, because neither Lisa nor anyone else could have met those needs. Certainly, Lisa believed it at first (because the pathological hope of the child was that if she'd just tried a bit harder, she'd have finally succeeded in getting him to love her). Finally, she began to examine their relationship and face the fact that her partner was incapable of love and that her constant pleasing was the only glue that had kept them together.

Lisa had been soothing her frustrations with comfort food and her partner had been increasingly critical of her weight. On a few occasions before he walked out, her resentment toward her partner overflowed and she couldn't resist lashing out at him in anger, which made him all the more rejecting. Once Lisa realized how her niceness and willingness to tolerate disrespect had backfired, she was ready to start looking at her own wounds and to work on healing them directly, rather than through being a pleaser.

Being nice and avoiding confrontation aren't the same as being loving and kind. Kindness, generosity, and altruism arise from adult concern for others. As I said before in the section on happiness, loving kindness comes out of a realization that we're all connected and responsible for the welfare of those in our community. This includes anything from feeding the birds in the winter to helping an elderly person cross a busy intersection, or stopping when someone has fallen on the sidewalk to help them up.

Loving kindness is standing up in the bus to let an elderly person sit down or holding a door open for a mother with a stroller. It's volunteering at the local animal shelter or helping feed the homeless. None of these actions are done to bring the doer love, but because they're helpful to others and because it feels good to be part of a community. An adult is kind and giving because she understands that she belongs to a greater whole and that when everyone participates in supporting each other, it strengthens the bonds of the community.

An adult doesn't begrudge energy spent on others. The child within doesn't resent it when we're kind to others because she's receiving the same loving kindness from the adult. Self-love fills a person up so that there's an overflow of love. Overflowing love doesn't deplete the giver, because it's a surplus of the love a person is already generating for herself. Also, because it doesn't deprive the giver of anything, the receiver never has to feel obligated.

This type of giving is the cleanest, healthiest way of being good to others and won't foster resentment. Instead of the child within trying to please others to "earn" love, the adult is sharing with others the love she has for her child within. Loving kindness brings happiness and contentment to the giver because it connects her with her community and makes her feel meaningfully engaged, whereas being nice results in feelings of frustration and resentment.

When an adult takes responsibility for loving and healing the child within, the child will no longer have to be in the forefront, seeking these things from others. The child will take her proper place in the background of the psyche and the adult will be free to let in the genuine affection of those who love her for herself. In participating in your community, experiencing self-love, and enjoying the no-strings-attached type of love with others, you'll be filled with the sort of positive feelings that are an antidote to overeating.

YOUR INNER WARRIOR

Maeve, a 48-year-old schoolteacher, was having a problem with a colleague at work. This other woman had a habit of speaking to her in a very rude manner. One day, after several months of therapy, Maeve was able to turn to this woman and say, "I'm sure you didn't intend to be as rude to me as you've been sounding." This stopped the woman in her tracks and she was never rude to Maeve again.

Eloise recently described an incident with a colleague who shares her office. This man is generally very grouchy and occasionally even hostile to her. One day, when Eloise passed him a requisition for some work, he began to complain loudly. Eloise was able, after spending some months in therapy, to stand up to this man in a way that didn't further antagonize him but instead, deflated his attempts at bullying. Both these victories came from these women having discovered what I call their "inner warrior."

Being an adult doesn't only refer to being reasonable, responsible, practical, and in charge of your impulses, but also involves some other important qualities. Just as the psyche can be theoretically divided into three parts, the adult part has a few subpersonalities as well. For example, in every person there's the "wise one within," or the inner wisdom aspect of the adult self. This is the part of you that knows things intuitively. It's an excellent part to call on when you need to figure something out and your intellect is confused. The wise part of you will guide you along the right path if you choose to listen to it. This part is the internalization of all the wise people the child encountered while she was growing up, and perhaps even an unconscious connection to the wisdom of all living things.

The aspect of the adult self that Maeve and Eloise developed in the previous examples is the *inner warrior,* and this part of the psyche is present in all living beings. Imagine how a mother bear would react if something threatened her cub. This, ideally, is how a human parent would act in response to any threat to her child. The inner warrior is the internalization of all the fierce and loving protection the child experienced from her caretakers, who are a child's first outer warriors. The inner warrior is strong to the degree that the child's parents or guardians defended and protected her. If the child was poorly protected or totally unprotected, she'll have a weak or absent inner warrior due to a lack of these outer role models.

The function of an inner warrior is to protect your child within from anything hurtful or dangerous, both externally and internally. In the outer world, its purpose is to identify and respond to any potentially dangerous or destructive person or situation. If the warrior part of the psyche isn't functioning well or at all, you aren't going to be able to tell what's safe and what's not, and you won't be able to take proper care of yourself. The inner warrior is also responsible for recognizing and combating the negative messages of the internalized parent, so if the warrior part of your psyche is weak or absent, the child within will be unprotected from the destructive messages of the inner critic.

If you were unprotected as a child and as a result, have a weak or absent inner warrior, you'll feel more vulnerable in the world and within yourself. Without a strong inner warrior, you'll be unable to develop the *self-trust* that comes from knowing you'll be able to defend the child within from internal or external onslaughts. A lack of self-trust creates anxiety because you can't rely on yourself. You'll have to find other ways of feeling safe, stuffing down your anxiety with food, hiding behind extra weight, withdrawing from intimate relationships, or being hypervigilant for potential danger.

Having an inner warrior is absolutely essential for getting through life without feeling overly vulnerable or unsafe. No one is completely safe in this world but with a warrior present, you're the safest you can be, as the warrior will be alert and aware of any danger. If it recognizes a potentially bad situation, the warrior will enable you to take action to either remove yourself, defend yourself, or get help from others, whichever is most appropriate.

Without the self-trust that comes from a strong inner warrior, it might be difficult for you to lose weight if you use the extra weight as a substitute for the warrior's protection. Having an inner warrior means being confident enough to feel that, "no matter what, I can handle what life throws me because I trust myself." If, in the absence of a strong inner warrior, you use your weight as a shield, it will be very hard for you to feel secure. This could lead to further weight gain in the unconscious hope that, eventually, you might feel "safe enough."

In the absence of the warrior, the child within is constantly at risk of being assaulted by the internalized parent. This parental part of the psyche, when unchecked, can turn into an inner critic, opponent, or even a killer, as its messages grow more destructive and undermine your self-worth and your motivation. It's crucial that the inner warrior be brought to bear against the inner opponent. If not, the child within will be forever at war with this destructive psychic force. The ongoing conflict will prevent the child from taking a back seat in the psyche and will interfere with the ability of the adult self to deal with the wounds that are driving the child to overeat. It's only when the inner warrior is present that the child within can feel safe enough to let the adult self take charge. It's only then that the adult can begin the process of self-healing and self-nurturing that will eliminate the need to overeat.

You might know or even be someone whose parents made her feel all turned around while she was growing up. She'd try, as a young child, to express what she was feeling to her parents but was either ignored or contradicted. This made her doubt her emotional reality and eventually, she became confused about what she was feeling and perceiving.

Being acknowledged as a child makes you grow up confident in your perceptions. You trust what you see, feel, and know and you're sure of yourself.

On the other hand, being told that you're wrong to have certain feelings, or hearing that you're not sad, hurt, or angry when you really do feel that way is very confusing. It can make you feel insecure, disconnected from yourself, and even unsure of what's real. This is why the inner warrior is so necessary. It's the antidote to parental or societal "crazy-making." It recognizes and rejects the confusing messages you're hearing and affirms that what you know and what you feel are real.

Fortunately, there are ways to develop an inner warrior even if you grew up without parents or caretakers who modeled this to you. One very helpful technique for developing different aspects of the psyche is a process called guided visualization. In the overeating workshops I lead, one of the first things we do is the visualization of "meeting the child within." Soon afterward, we do a visualization introducing the group members to the inner warrior.

VISUALIZATION 2: MEETING THE INNER WARRIOR

Again, sitting comfortably on a straight-backed chair in a quiet room with your shoes, glasses, and watch removed, bring your attention to your breathing. Let your breaths come easily and in slow and steady inhalations and exhalations. Plant your feet on the floor, and let the chair and the floor support your body so that you can settle down and begin to relax. Close your eyes and find yourself once again in the small, cozy room, sitting on the beautiful, comfortable chair. Notice the small door directly in front of you, the full-length mirror in the ornate gilded frame on the wall to the right of the door, the small round window high up on the wall to the left of the door, and the three tall urns on the floor against the wall below the window.

Bring your attention to the small door in front of you and notice that it's beginning to open. The child within is entering the room. Don't be surprised if she's not the same child as you've met on other occasions. In this visualization, you can meet the child at any of her ages and stages, depending on what your psyche needs to work on at the moment. Try to embrace whichever version of the child it is who walks through the door.

Invite her to come and sit in the chair with you and this time, insist that she does for her own safety and comfort. Then, when the child is comfortably sitting beside you or in your lap, bring your attention to the mirror on the wall. Notice that the reflective part of the mirror is beginning to fill with smoke from the edges of the frame inward, and that the smoke is starting to swirl around within the frame. As the smoke swirls, a space is beginning to clear in the center of the mirror, and the smoke is now retreating to the corners of the frame. Finally, it disappears, but this time, it leaves only the frame, and an open space where the mirror used to be.

As you look at the space within the frame, you see a long tunnel extending far back. A figure is walking toward you, approaching the edge of the frame. It's your inner warrior. Observe if it's male or female, human or animal, a real or mythical creature. It might be frightening to look at but remember that this is *your* inner warrior, here to protect and defend the child within you, so you need not fear it. Notice what you feel as the warrior steps into the room.

Invite the warrior to come and stand in front of you. Pay attention to how the child is reacting to the ~~~~~~~~~ us, reassure her, but often,
the varrior within, because she
unc from now on. Begin to talk
wit ything to say to you. Listen
clo r being there for you and
the

war ou communicate with the
You to be part of you forever.
spa he small room, but there's
to g to stand. Ask the warrior
Nov warrior "has your back."
you it's standing behind you,
enei rning into a column of
Feel ry pulsating behind you.
mer o move toward you and
noti your entire spine and
inne it you have a sense of

N reaction to the warrior
havii to shimmer, glimmer,
and l st, and feel her entering yo Sit in your beautiful,
comfo ur spine and the child
energy be so connected with
these t o reality carrying the
child a you. Know that you can go back to this room any time to connect with the inner warrior.

Another powerful way of developing the inner warrior is by using role models in your adult life. Being in a long-term therapeutic relationship can help you develop an inner warrior by seeing how a warrior operates in the world. The therapist is a model for her clients or patients in how she takes care of herself, and can demonstrate to you warrior-like qualities, especially in areas such as the maintenance of healthy boundaries. How the therapist treats you is the other important way you can learn to develop an inner warrior. By caring about your well-being, working on your behalf for your healing and growth, and supporting your empowerment in the face of your inner and outer opponents, your therapist can model to you what, perhaps, your parents couldn't. This can help you learn how to protect and defend yourself.

Another model for an inner warrior can come from anyone in your life who's stood up for you or who's taken your side when you needed an advocate. It could be a teacher, doctor, coach, family member, or friend. It could be a member of the clergy or even a relative stranger. The experience of having someone who's there for you shows you that it's normal to expect protection and defense as a child, that you are entitled to these things and that self-defense is both necessary and possible.

There are also many models of the warrior in literature and in the media to draw inspiration from: whether it's *Xena: Warrior Princess,* one of the noble warriors in *The Lord of the Rings,* Uma Thurman's character in the movie *Kill Bill,* a Samurai soldier, a Masai warrior, Yoda of *Star Wars* fame, a Greek god, or Wonder Woman, there's no shortage of figures to draw upon for your inner warrior. These models are all fierce fighters, and demonstrate what it means to stand up against the forces of darkness, destructiveness, or oppression.

Even if you had no one there to protect or defend you when you were young, by making use of your therapist or any other warrior model, you can come to see that being protected and defended is crucial if you're to feel safe and secure. You can develop your own inner warrior that can then combat the destructive, undermining attacks of the inner opponent, and stand up to any external threats to your safety, security, or self-worth.

It's important to note that the inner warrior is a powerful fighter but its role is not to do harm or commit acts of violence. The inner warrior is a psychological tool that you'll use in becoming empowered. Having a strong inner warrior is about being well protected and defended, as opposed to hostile and aggressive. The inner warrior enables you to be calmly assertive through the self-trust it gives you. Someone with the confidence of the inner warrior has nothing to prove and doesn't need to make a big noise in order to take care of herself. Someone connected with their inner warrior is quietly secure instead of noisily defensive. Bullies and blowhards lack inner warriors and are compensating by trying to dominate or control others.

THE TRUTH ABOUT FORGIVING

My patient Moira came to me one day with a dilemma. She'd been reading a lot of self-help books telling her to forgive the people who had caused her harm or she'd never be healed. She began to cry, saying that she wanted to heal but that she just couldn't forgive her parents, who'd emotionally abused her as a child. She was torn because she believed what these books were saying, but she couldn't bring herself to forgive what to her were unforgivable acts of cruelty. Fortunately for Moira, the books were wrong and she didn't have to forgive her parents for what they did in order to heal the wounds of her childhood.

Some people are convinced that they need to forgive their parents—or any other people who might have hurt them—as part of the healing process. They think that with forgiveness, they'll be able to let go of the past and to move on. I don't agree with this. It's been my experience that *healing requires letting go* of old wounds, but that *forgiveness isn't required* in order to let go. Forcing yourself to forgive because you've been told by a book, a parent, or an authority figure that it's the "right" thing to do might actually reinforce your wounds because you're trying to make yourself do something that, deep down, doesn't feel right to you.

Some people find it easy and natural to forgive, but it's not like this for everyone. If it doesn't feel right, making yourself forgive someone who's done something terrible to you feels like you're betraying yourself. The internalized parent is telling you that you "should" be able to forgive them, when in your heart and soul, you really can't. The good news is that you don't need to forgive, either for moral reasons or for your healing.

Some acts are simply unforgivable. I've observed people trying to force themselves to forgive the unforgivable and they become increasingly upset with themselves when they can't do it. I've seen people racked with shame and guilt because they were convinced that to be a good person, they needed to forgive.

So many of our institutions and leaders promote the ideal of forgiveness, but I suspect that in part, it might be a way for those in our society who've hurt us or disappointed us to get away with being thoughtless or destructive, because they've taught us that we must forgive. The perpetrators of harm benefit from being forgiven, but it doesn't necessarily help the victims. Forgiving those who hurt us often allows the perpetrators to continue being hurtful, and the victims to continue to be hurt.

I see another way of addressing this issue. Rather than forcing yourself to forgive, you can simply let go. The process of conscious grieving will enable you to release the wounds of the past as much as you believed forgiveness would. Grieving and letting go will make it possible for you to release any residual hurt, anger, fear, or helplessness and will cleanly detach you from those who've wronged you. You'll have no unfinished business with anybody once you've fully grieved and let go, and you'll carry no leftover emotions. You'll find a sense of peace and relief from this process of facing, grieving, and letting go that you'd never discover by trying to force yourself to forgive.

The grieving process facilitates freedom and empowerment, but forcing yourself to forgive can create guilt, shame, and confusion as the internalized parent keeps telling the child within that she should do something she simply can't. I see forgiveness as optional and dependent on certain circumstances. Some actions, as I said, are unforgivable. For example, I could never forgive Hitler and his followers for the atrocities they committed. In the case of forgivable things, like carelessness, insensitivity, or selfishness, it's my opinion that it might be appropriate to forgive the responsible individual(s) under the following circumstances; what I call "doing the right thing."

If the person who committed the hurtful act acknowledges his mistake to you; if he committed the act out of his own unconscious wounds rather than maliciously and deliberately in order to cause harm; if he understands how it hurt you and is truly remorseful; if he apologizes sincerely for what he's done and promises never to repeat the act; if he follows through on this promise and doesn't repeat the hurtful behavior; and if he makes amends for having hurt you, then, if it feels right to you, you may be comfortable with forgiving him. It won't have any effect on your healing, but it will enable you to maintain a better, more open relationship with the other person if you choose to do so.

If the other person won't do the right thing, you'll still be able to heal your wounds by facing the truth about how they hurt you and by grieving and letting go of your wounds. Knowing that this other person wouldn't acknowledge the hurtful act, apologize, or change their behavior will provide you with important information about him: either he has no remorse, has committed his act deliberately or maliciously, is in denial about his behavior, doesn't care enough about you to apologize and make amends, or is unwilling to take responsibility for the harm he's done.

Having this information is empowering because it helps you to see that without remorse or the desire to change, this person is likely to reoffend. It will quickly become clear that it's preferable for you to avoid someone who takes no responsibility for his hurtfulness and who's highly likely to hurt you again.

Forgiving someone who hasn't done the right thing has a number of consequences. First of all, it puts you in an unsafe situation. Second, forgiving might make you believe that you've healed and that you're a good person, but it sets up an inner conflict between the internalized parent, who says you must forgive, and the child within, who doesn't want to do this.

Forgiveness isn't freeing or empowering, whereas letting go through grieving and taking good care of the child within is. Some people might ask, "but what about the anger you'll be holding on to if you don't forgive?" They've missed the point. Facing how you've been hurt, grieving your losses, letting them go, and lovingly caring for the child within will free you of any residual hurt, anger, fear, or sadness you've been carrying. Facing and grieving your losses is the way to completely let go of the past and a far better solution to having been hurt by someone than forgiveness ever will be. Plus, it has the benefit of preventing you from being hurt again by these people in the future.

CELESTE'S STORY

Not long ago, I worked with a woman named Celeste, who'd come into therapy after becoming involved with an abusive man. At the beginning of the relationship he'd been charming and attentive and he made her feel "like a princess." Soon, however, she began to see that he was controlling, critical, aggressive, unreasonable, and intolerant of her. He began to behave more and more badly, all the while complaining to her that it was she who was disappointing him. She could no longer tolerate his behavior and after some time, finally left him, at which point he became so enraged that he began to stalk and harass her. She came to therapy to work on her overeating issues, but quickly it became clear that first she needed to address the relationship issues that were driving her to overeat.

Celeste's ex-partner lacked the capacity for real love or empathy, and was driven to exploit the women he was with. Celeste was new to therapy and had come in with deep wounds from childhood that she hadn't begun to heal. She admitted that she'd seen her ex as someone who'd bring her fulfillment and take away her pain. In Celeste's eyes, her ex had represented the end to her loneliness and a way of finally being loved; something she'd never had from her parents. She'd been convinced that being with this man was the way that she could feel better about herself.

Celeste's partner was ultimately shown to be cold and manipulative, extremely self-centered, entitled, and exploitative. He was contemptuous of society's rules and unable to truly love, have empathy, or experience remorse. Like all predatory people, he was highly attuned to the signs of emotional wounds in others. He quickly recognized Celeste's neediness and charmed her into thinking that he cared. He took advantage of her infatuation by getting her to support him financially and tolerate his bad behavior.

One thing that exploitative men (or women) are looking for in a partner is to take advantage of their desperation. The predatory man knows that a desperate woman sees him as the answer to her needs and therefore will have a hard time leaving him. He understands that for this reason, she'll have a very high tolerance for his controlling, neglectful, or even abusive behavior so he doesn't hold back on any of it once he's sure that the woman is "hooked."

If the child within has chosen to be with a man because she's convinced that he's her salvation, it's because the woman has abdicated her adult power and allowed the child to be emotionally dependent on the man. He'll take advantage of this dependency by getting everything he can out of the woman. The child within believes that it's better to stay with this hurtful man than to be alone, so she'll accept behavior from him that a self-sufficient adult would never tolerate.

Celeste had become addicted to the fantasy of love from her partner and for a long time was unable to extricate herself from the relationship. The child within her held onto the pathological hope that if she were to stay with this man long enough, then eventually her wounds would be healed and her need for love and nurturing would be met. She didn't want to face the fact that he didn't love her and in fact, was behaving more and more badly toward her.

An abusive, exploitative partner looks for someone who's desperate, needy, and willing to give up her power and autonomy. What he also looks for is the woman's *willingness to deny that he's bad.* Celeste saw her man not as a potentially dangerous predator, incapable of caring for her, but as a wounded little boy who needed her care to transform him into a loving man. This denial of dangerousness played into the man's agenda and enabled him to continue his bad behavior.

Celeste was willing to see him as troubled but not as dangerous, because she so desperately wanted a surrogate parent to take care of her emotional needs. When a woman (or man) gets involved with a predator, it's almost always because the person has presented himself or herself as someone who'll meet those needs for her or him. Men like Celeste's ex use their charm and cunning to convince women that they're caring and giving, as opposed to what they really are: cold-blooded users and abusers.

People who repeatedly choose to be with charming users can be said to be addicted to love, because they have a very hard time facing the truth about the destructive nature of these relationships and an even harder time letting them go. They're using the relationships in the same way as an overeater uses food: to heal emotional wounds and meet emotional needs. The infatuation they feel is really just the pathological hope of the child, burning within them. They'll have had a string of such hurtful relationships because they're compelled, like any other addict, to repeat the behavior until it finally pays off. Love addiction is just as unfulfilling and at least as destructive as any other addiction.

Interestingly, the woman who goes for a predatory man is attracted to him, in part, because he reminds her of the people she sought love from in the past and, in part, because they share similar wounds. The difference is that they're opposite sides of the same coin. Where she takes the passive, victim role, he takes the active, abuser role.

These predatory men have within them the same wounded child that the woman has and are trying to compensate for childhood hurts and losses in their own, dysfunctional way. Sadly, they're as unsuccessful as anyone else who's looking outside himself for the answer to his suffering. These men are compelled to dominate, control, and exploit the other person in an attempt to fulfill their persistent needs, but because outer solutions are inadequate for addressing inner wounds, these men are left frustrated.

The woman who's addicted to love sees the wounded child hidden within her man. The wounded part of her identifies with this child and she naively wants to help heal the child within the man. She intuitively recognizes how needy this man really is, and believes that if she just loves and cares for him enough, he'll be grateful and will eventually give her love. It's a throwback to her belief in childhood that loving her (wounded, hurtful) parents enough would get them to finally love her back.

She forgets that her partner express his neediness not in the clingy, dependent ways that she does, but in hurtful, aggressive, even violent behavior. She doesn't want to see that although he might have a wounded, needy little boy within, his behavior in the real world is that of a dangerous, fully grown man.

Unfortunately, in the world of adults, the only people who are able to take on the role of the "good parent" with no strings attached are actual parents. The emotional and physical demands of parenting are so great that an ordinary person would never want to care for anyone but their own beloved child (exceptions being a sick, elderly, or disabled loved one, or a pet). When, apart from a professional relationship (such as a nurse, doctor, counselor, or cleric), one adult is willing to take on the care of another who's able-bodied, able-minded, and fully capable of self-care, it's clear that the caretaker must have ulterior motives.

Of course, there are both male and female predators, and two men or two women together can play out any of the previous roles. Since my book is primarily geared to women who overeat, I'm focusing on the women who get involved with these types of men because of how it relates to their particular issues, especially with regard to eating and weight.

A nonprofessional who'll take on the care of a fully grown, otherwise competent adult is one who has something to gain by entering into such an arrangement. A more benign version of a caretaker is the emotionally needy man who'll get into a relationship with a needy woman, with the proviso that there's reciprocity and she'll, in turn, care for him. For a while she can be the child and he can be the "daddy," and then he gets to be the child, and she must take on the "mommy" role. If a woman goes along with this arrangement, she'll be entering into a codependent relationship in which, for at least 50 percent of the time, she'll be someone's surrogate mother.

That's a high price to pay for being able to be the child the rest of the time, but many women initially go along with this arrangement. The dynamic doesn't work, though, in the long run. While the woman is in the caretaking role, she resents her position and would rather be in the cared-for role. She feels burdened and frustrated by the selfish and unreasonable demands of her partner while he's taking his turn as the child in the relationship. On the other hand, when she finally gets to be the child, she ends up just as resentful because being controlled and infantilized is frustrating and humiliating to her.

In codependency, neither person gets to enjoy each other as adults where they could see the best in each other. In fact, this type of relationship brings out the worst in each person: the nagging, bossy, critical parent, or the overwhelmed, helpless, demanding child. Both sides of the equation resent their roles, feeling either burdened or belittled. Both can't help but express their anger at each other, usually indirectly, because neither can be open with his anger due to a childlike fear of abandonment.

This creates a potentially toxic situation where each partner will tolerate the things in the relationship that bother them, rather than be abandoned, but neither one can avoid leaking their anger at the other. The passive-aggressive behavior creates a vicious circle because one partner's indirectly expressed anger causes the other partner to be angry, too, which increases the existing level of resentment. When both partners fear abandonment and both exhibit passive-aggressive behaviors, the level of buried hostility between them increases until, inevitably, there's an explosion and a temporary or permanent rupture of the relationship.

In codependency, both participants are pursuing addiction in the form of a relationship. Both are driven by the most self-centered, needy aspect of the child within. Neither one of them is taking responsibility for him-or-herself and neither is really capable of caring about his or her partner. Codependency is the shared addiction of two children in a relationship. Each one is using the other for love and healing. Until they can no longer stand it, they continue to hope that this will be the answer for them.

Addiction to love is as obsessive and compulsive as any other addiction. The person is compelled to stay in a bad relationship out of pathological hope. She's obsessed with how she can get her partner to love her and heal the wounds of her childhood and she's compelled to keep trying to make it work, even when it's not working for her.

Women who look for healing in their relationship have a lot in common with women who overeat: the main thing they share is a history of significant childhood losses or trauma and a deep wish to be the loved and nurtured child. Both food-addicted and love-addicted women are driven by the needy child within who's convinced that these external solutions will heal her wounds and meet her needs. Whether as a compulsive overeater or someone who compulsively pursues a dysfunctional relationship, a woman who looks for healing anywhere but from within herself is inadvertently creating a vicious circle of disappointment and repeated attempts at meeting her needs through the addiction.

If a woman has an addiction to love as well as an overeating problem (which is not uncommon, seeing as how they both have the same source), her compulsive attempts to get someone to love her will end up also supporting her compulsive eating behavior. As she tries in vain to have this person compensate for the love she didn't receive while growing up, and as they refuse to do this for her, she'll be compelled to seek comfort through overeating instead. The more Celeste became frustrated in her relationship, the more she began to stuff down her feelings with food. She gained 50 pounds in the 2 years she and her partner were together.

Freedom for a woman with food and love addictions will come in the form of embracing her adult identity and in taking responsibility for healing and nurturing the child within. When a woman can be there for herself, she'll no longer be a slave to addiction. This means letting go of the child role, and especially the victim role.

The victim role is an aspect of the child, the way the warrior is an aspect of the adult self. The victim feels like she's been hurt, wronged, and hard done by. She's the "adult child" of an alcoholic; the "survivor" of abuse or trauma. This is her primary identity, more than any other role she inhabits in her adult life. She's overly invested in seeing herself as wounded and in need of compensation for her wounds. The world owes her caretaking and healing because of how much she's suffered.

Of course, her trauma and suffering are real, but these don't have to define her. By identifying herself as a victim, a woman can never escape this role and she'll live her adult life being the wounded child, pursuing child-like solutions to her wounds. She'll also continue being exploited and victimized by others, because if she walks around letting everyone know that she feels like a victim, others will gladly collude with her. If she abdicates responsibility for her self-care, there will always be predators around who will offer her the false promises of rescue.

A woman will never break free of her addictions if she remains in the victim role because it's a passive state in which she blames everyone else for her pain and suffering. It's always everyone else's fault when a woman is a victim and because of this, she's powerless to affect positive change on her own behalf. As a result, she'll continue to suffer without respite.

There's a belief held by many people that's detrimental to their welfare. This belief is that psychotherapy or any other form of counseling is either unnecessary or useless. Thinking this way often prevents people from solving the problems in their lives that are causing them unhappiness or suffering. A number of my patients over the years have said to me: "I've always believed that I should be able to sort it all out by myself." These people felt ashamed that they needed help from a therapist to deal with their wounds.

I explained the same thing to each of them: the internalized parent was telling them the lie that they "should" be able to heal their wounds without help. The perfectionist, unreasonable parental voice in their head was placing unfair expectations on these individuals and making them feel bad for needing assistance in their healing process. In reality, it's very hard to completely overcome anxiety, depression, neuroses, or addictions without professional support. Some people turn to friends for support, thinking that this is less "shameful" than seeking professional help. Friends are wonderful and have the best intentions, but they give advice that's often biased and not helpful, and sometimes even counterproductive.

It's a built-in survival mechanism for the psyche to resist change. Any movement toward change in your beliefs or behavior patterns will tend to cause you discomfort or stress. We're creatures of habit, even when our habits are harmful. It's also unlikely that a person could have the necessary objectivity and skill required to fully heal her own emotional wounds. A caring, experienced professional can be extremely helpful in empowering a person to overcome her internal resistance to change, heal her wounds, and develop self-love. Good therapy, far from being "useless," is an invaluable resource for personal growth.

It's essential for you to be familiar with the steps in the healing process, but this isn't always enough for you to fully succeed in your healing. Once you've become aware that you have wounds (perhaps because you've realized that you have eating habits and weight that are out of control), then you need to know that *you don't have to do it all by yourself.* I recommend a therapist who has enough training, experience, and ruthless compassion to be comfortable and confident guiding you through the course of your healing.

She can help you face the past without fear or denial, and she can help support you as you go into the process of grieving your childhood losses. A good therapist should be the warrior for consciousness and empowerment on your behalf, and should show you how to battle the demons of helplessness, hopelessness, victimhood, self-blame, guilt, shame, and self-hatred. The therapist should help you develop a strong adult identity, enable you to identify and reject the negativity of outer opponents and the internalized parent, and help you begin to love, support, heal, and protect the child within.

In my mind, the ideal therapist is a psychological midwife, facilitating the emergence of the most authentic, fully realized, and optimal version of you.

A good therapist walks with you through the painful valley of the past, with all its dark secrets. She helps you shine light on hidden truths and enables you to confront them with strength and courage. She models wholeness and empowerment so that you may emerge from your journey as an intact, fully functioning adult.

The therapist will help you to remember that you might *have* a child within, but you *aren't* the child within. The therapeutic process will help you stop identifying with this child, and will remind you that you're an intelligent, resourceful, resilient grown-up who is absolutely strong enough to tolerate any emotion that might arise out of the process of facing the past. Therapy will support you in recognizing that you've already lived through these painful emotions and survived them when you were smaller, weaker, and less resourceful than you are today. With those experiences behind you, you'll come to see that since you've already survived every emotion you went through as a child, it stands to reason that you'll be able to tolerate them and use them for your healing now as an adult.

Some people fear crying, believing that if they start, they'll never stop. Some feel that crying means that they're weak, self-indulgent, or full of self-pity. This is the message of the internalized parent and it's untrue. Crying from a conscious place of grieving real losses is courageous, because it's associated with facing painful truths and letting go of old wounds. Therapy will reinforce the fact that crying is really an act of self-love. Shedding tears is an essential part of the healing process. Your therapist will support you in your grieving by being a solid, secure adult presence and by empowering you to be there for your child within.

The healing process is also about connecting with other feelings. Anger is a significant emotion that needs to be dealt with but which might be frightening to experience alone. As I mentioned previously, if the child has grown up in an environment in which anger was inappropriately expressed and where she became frightened or even horrified by the way anger was used, it's likely that she'll be afraid of her own anger, believing that it will be as destructive as the anger of her childhood.

The child's first experience of other people's anger will permanently color her impression of this emotion, until such time as she has the opportunity to see it in a different light. While the child within is still seeing anger as something destructive or dangerous, she'll have difficulty facing the anger she's carrying toward the people who hurt or disappointed her when she was growing up. The child's anger will get bottled up in response to her fear that it will be as hurtful to her or to others as the anger she experienced in the past. She'd rather stuff the anger down or direct it inward, than risk being just like those who hurt her. Your therapist can help you deal with your anger in a constructive and positive way.

Anger that's bottled up is a strong motivating factor for overeating because a very effective way of temporarily stuffing down unwanted emotion is by stuffing yourself with food. Since it's only a short-term solution, the act has to be repeated over and over again to keep this forbidden emotion from surfacing. It's clear, then, that dealing with your anger from childhood will be very helpful in overcoming compulsive eating.

Anger can be healed in a different way than pain, hurt, and feelings of loss. Anger is a more active type of emotion and needs action to help it come out. The child within might be afraid to express her held-in anger, especially if she's kept it in for a long time. It might feel like there's a volcano inside her that's ready to erupt, and it might seem that she could hurt someone if she were to let this volcano blow. In a safe, controlled therapeutic environment, your therapist can help you access these feelings without becoming overwhelmed and remind you that as an adult, you're in charge of your impulses and emotional expression and that nothing bad is going to happen if you feel your anger.

EXERCISES FOR THE CONSTRUCTIVE RELEASE OF ANGER

There are simple, constructive exercises you can do to help access and release buried anger. You can take paper and crayons and draw pictures of your angry feelings. You could write an angry letter to the person or people who you feel have hurt you. (The letters aren't meant to be sent. This is not an exercise in confronting others, but one for releasing pent-up emotion.) You could go for a run, or bat a ball around with a racket.

If you're alone, and the walls are fairly soundproof, here's a suggestion for releasing deep-seated rage: pile up a bunch of cushions on the floor and kneel in front of them. Visualize in your mind's eye the person or people who you feel have hurt you the most, and begin to punch the cushions and yell at the people. You can express how you feel about what they've done or you can just make a loud noise, or shout, "no!" "no more!" or "never again!" while you're punching the cushions. This might seem a bit extreme to you, but if you're sitting on years of held-in anger, it might be the only safe way your anger can come out.

Don't forget that no one is getting hurt with these exercises, and that it's preferable to yell and punch pillows than to make yourself fat by stuffing down your anger with food. Anger itself is not a "bad" emotion, but you might have learned the wrong message about it if you witnessed inappropriate expressions of anger when you were a child.

Doing these exercises will help you in a number of ways: you'll be able to see that anger is just a feeling like all the others, and that it's not necessarily destructive. In fact, you'll see that you need your anger because when you're afraid of it and don't let yourself feel it, you're at risk of not getting angry when you should and therefore not taking care of yourself. You'll learn that there's a time and a place for the appropriate expression of anger and that when it's not pent-up or seething just below the surface, you won't need to work so hard at stuffing it back in with food. When you can let your anger out in a healthy way, you won't have the social consequences of passive-aggressive behavior or inappropriate leaks of repressed anger. Finally, when you let go of your many years of held-in anger, your food cravings related to it will disappear.

If you use your therapy to support you in fully grieving the losses of your childhood and in releasing your residual hurt, pain, and anger, you'll get to the point where you'll start letting go of your wounds. Having mourned your losses, you'll no longer identify yourself as the victim of a bad childhood, because letting go of your wounds will have shifted your identity from that of a helpless child-victim to that of an empowered adult, free to pursue her true goals.

5

CARING FOR THE CHILD WITHIN YOU: EMPOWERED CHOICES FOR REAL HAPPINESS

Amelia is a normal-weight 45-year-old receptionist who recently admitted that she used to get on the scale every day, sometimes twice a day. It had become a compulsive behavior, driven by an obsession with her weight. She was compelled to keep weighing herself despite the fact that her weight changed very little from weigh-in to weigh-in. She couldn't understand why she had to do this.

Many women, whatever they weigh, share this problem with the scale. They obsess about every pound and have within them a parental voice that criticizes them for failing to "measure up." If this is you, the scale has become the outer representation of the internalized parent as it stares up you with constant reproach. You try and try to meet the weight that the scale (as parent) demands, but even if you do, you'll never be able to please it. Whether or not you're overweight, if you're compelled to check your weight repeatedly, you need to see that this is as much a compulsion as overeating is, and you must let it go. Otherwise, it will reinforce the power of the internalized parent and set up an inner struggle that you can never win.

The scale is not your friend. It promotes obsessive thinking about weight and compulsive self-weighing (and dieting) behavior. Even if you've lost all the weight you wanted to, constantly weighing yourself makes you a prisoner of the scale's tyranny. You don't need to obsess how much weight you're losing every day or every week or how much you weigh on a daily or weekly basis after the weight loss. Your body will show you. Being conscious of how your body feels and how your clothes fit are enough to tell you if you're going up or down in weight. Getting back into your old clothes or just feeling good and healthy in your body should be the goals of any new health regime. The scale won't help you lose weight but it will keep the obsessive and compulsive aspects of your eating issues front-and-center.

When you stand on the scale, the child sets herself up to be criticized for "failing" to succeed. The *obsession* with minute changes in weight comes from listening to the internalized parent's impossible demands and trying to please it. It perpetuates an addict's mind-set, as does the *compulsion* to weigh yourself constantly so as to make sure you're doing what the critic wants.

One behavioral intervention that will immediately decrease the obsessing and compulsiveness is to *get rid of your scale*. Toss it into the trash. If you're working to connect with the child within, heal your wounds and pursue your true needs, the weight will come off without the use of a scale. In the end, you'll know when your body feels right and how to eat to maintain a healthy weight without ever having to stand on a scale. You can be like anyone who doesn't have an eating and weight issue, getting weighed by your family doctor at your annual checkup. Let go of shame, self-blame, the obsessions, and compulsive behaviors and ditch the scale.

Molly was a tall, lively 42-year-old teacher who went into therapy because of a difficult situation. She simply couldn't lose weight. As therapy progressed, soon it became clear why not. Every time she tried to stop her after-dinner binges, her husband would bring home junk food after work and eat it in front of her. Molly didn't want to believe that the man she loved was sabotaging her plans to get healthy, but eventually, she could no longer deny it. Finally, he admitted that he was so used to the overweight Molly that he was terrified to encounter the stranger that the thin Molly would be to him. Out of his fear of change, he was doing his best to keep his wife overweight.

Amy, on the other hand, was a 50-something bookkeeper who came to therapy because she'd begin to lose weight and then plateau. She didn't understand why she could never go below a certain weight. In therapy, she realized that when her body really started to change, she began to develop an identity crisis with growing anxiety and confusion about who she was. Through therapy, she learned to separate the weight from who she really was and to see herself just as "Amy," as opposed to, "Amy the overweight woman."

If you've been overweight for a long time, it can become easy to identify yourself in this way. People are creatures of habit and tend to feel most secure when things remain stable and insecure when things change, even for the better. If you've been heavy for a long time, you and the people around you may have grown comfortable with you being that way. Some people in your life might even be invested in your being overweight for their own reasons, and some might feel uncomfortable or even threatened if you begin to lose weight.

After several years of carrying around extra weight, you can begin to believe that the real you is a heavy person. You might even forget the thinner person you used to be, becoming psychologically adapted to your new heavier self. Like Amy, you might become anxious when you begin to lose weight. The thought, "who am I now?" might go through your mind. You might ask yourself, "if I stop being heavy, who would I be?" These questions can be very upsetting as you begin losing weight. Weight loss might be a good idea theoretically, but in practice it can be overwhelming. If your friends, life partner, or family members are equally attached to the idea of you as a fat person, then it'll be that much more difficult for you to lose weight.

It's important that you understand two things: first, no matter how others see you or how they want to see you, *you own your body* and have the last word on what shape and size it should be. Some people might be pressuring you to be thin; others might need you to be heavy, but that shouldn't interfere with you becoming healthy or having the body that you really want.

Second, you can say to yourself, "I may be carrying fat, but *I am not my fat.*" Who you are has more to do with your heart and soul and much less with your size, which is only one aspect of you. What's most important is what's inside each person, so no matter how much weight you gain or lose, you never stop being yourself.

In Molly's case, she needed to reassure her husband that the only thing that was going to be different about her was her size, and that he wasn't going to lose the woman that he knew and loved if she were to lose weight.

If you've been working on healing your wounds and giving the child within what she needs, then eventually you'll be free of the dysfunctional child-based thinking and behavior patterns associated overeating and overweight and you'll lose the urge to eat the way you used to. The weight will begin to melt away, but even more importantly, being free of your obsessions and compulsions will represent a far more significant personality change than any amount of weight loss.

Not everyone with a weight problem has been heavy since childhood. Some men might have begun to gain weight during high school or college; some women might do so at puberty, after the birth of a child, or in middle age. Although it's true that emotional needs and wounds drive overeating and weight gain, sometimes a woman will have a very resilient personality and her childhood hurts or losses won't affect her immediately. Sometimes, a woman can get lucky in her adult life, where everything is going well and the wounds of the past aren't going to affect her as strongly.

In everyone's life, though, bad things happen. If you were someone who's experienced childhood hurts or losses, but managed to get away with living a life free of compulsive eating for many years, all it would have taken was a *stressor* to tip you over the edge and into compulsive overeating and weight gain. A stressor is anything that causes your wounds to rise to the surface and trigger the child within to pursue her agenda of healing and compensating for her losses.

It could happen during puberty, when dating becomes an issue, or in college when you're transitioning into adulthood. It can happen when you go from being your parents' child to being a mother or when you experience the pain of romantic rejection. Any of these stressors can upset the balance you'd originally achieved between your wounds and resilience, and can cause you to develop the eating disorder that had been dormant. Maybe you had some unusual eating habits beforehand, but now you've become a full-fledged binge eater.

It takes a while to adjust your sense of self from the previously average-weight person you used to be to the now overweight person you've become.

As creatures of habit, our identity is something we're very reluctant to relinquish. It can be painful to let go of a slim self-image as in our society, this is associated with being attractive. Adopting a "less-attractive," overweight self-image is a blow to the ego.

It's important to note that it takes just as much of an adjustment when you lose a significant amount of weight as when you've gained it. You'd think that it would be easy to let go of this "less-desirable" self-image but in fact, any major change is uncomfortable for most people. If you've spent years being overweight, your size has become almost inseparable from your identity. Letting go of that familiar, comfortable identity can be as stressful as it was for the woman who had to get used to being heavy after years of being thin.

It's hard enough to make this shift in identity, but if you're attached to pleasing everyone else and afraid of their potential negative reactions to your changed physique, the adjustment will be that much more difficult. If, on the other hand, you're comfortable in the knowledge that you're always yourself regardless of your size and not subject to the reactions of your loved ones, then the adjustment will be easier. In reality, no one is a static being. We're always changing and growing, adapting and recreating ourselves, and yet fundamentally we're always still ourselves. Just think for a moment about yourself as a 5-year-old. Don't you have the same likes, dislikes, and personality you had then? The important question is: will you let anything stop you from being the best version of yourself that you can be?

There's another issue involved with body image, and it's especially true for women. It's the fear you might have of being as attractive, powerful, and successful as you could be. You might develop this fear if a parent was threatened by or resented the beauty or talent you exhibited while growing up. It could also result from having been made to feel guilty for surpassing a jealous parent in any area. You might feel the need to play down your appearance or any other gifts so as not to incite parental displeasure and possible rejection.

It's conceivable that you could have gained weight to become less threatening to your parent(s). This is particularly common if you've grown up with a narcissistic parent who resented her child for doing better or having more than she did in life. As an adult, you might remain heavy so as not to be competition to your female peers. Maybe you've chosen friends who are similar to your parents. These jealous friends could resent your good looks and imply that they'll reject you if you become "too attractive." Even if your friends aren't like this, you might still believe, based on past experience that your friends are as challenged by your attributes as your parents have been.

As a young girl, you might have noticed your father, another male relative, or a teacher looking at your body with an interest that made you feel uncomfortable or even dirty. Even if he didn't act on his inappropriate feelings, his staring would have been enough to give you the wrong message about your appearance. You'd begin to feel that your body was dangerous, seductive, and something that could get you into trouble, so you might then feel the need to neutralize your sexual attractiveness by hiding it under a lot of weight.

There may be many reasons why a woman could grow up feeling uncomfortable with her beauty or sexual attractiveness. If you've developed an unconscious or even deliberate habit of downplaying your appearance, it can be difficult to break. This behavior is connected to your primal fears of maternal abandonment, paternal violation, or too-early sexuality. It might even have been reinforced by parental messages that it's wrong to show off or attract the attention of men.

Overcoming a habit of gaining weight in order to downplay your attractiveness requires the presence of an inner warrior. The confidence the warrior brings enables you to see that as an adult, you no longer need your mother's approval; you no longer need to fear the jealousy of a friend or your father's— or any man's—gaze. A powerful inner warrior enables you to trust your own capacity for self-care so that other peoples' needs or expectations are no longer your focus. In this way, you're free to be your best, most attractive self.

With a powerful inner warrior, a woman can be as beautiful and sensual in her body as she chooses. Having a strong warrior means that you'll be protected from competition, disapproval, rejection, or inappropriate attention. In every situation, the alert warrior will tell you what's going on and show you what you need to do to be safe and sound. A child can't stand up for herself and is unable to walk away from a bad situation. With a well-developed inner warrior, you'll be able to do both of these things as an adult.

Having a powerful inner warrior hones your powers of observation so that you can assess every situation critically and then determine whether it's safe or appropriate for you. The inner warrior pays attention to the people with whom you're associating and takes action when necessary to protect you from harm. The child within you acts out of wishful thinking, ignoring, or denying any signals that might indicate the potential for emotional danger. She deludes herself, convinced that she'll be safe hiding behind the weight, or other dysfunctional defenses. The warrior, on the other hand, alerts you to these danger signals, enabling you to act on them in order to be truly safe without the need for the false protection of the extra weight.

With these reality based tools, you can develop trust in your own perceptions and the confidence to act on what's actually happening around you. You won't need to hide your beauty, sexual power, or sensuality behind a wall of extra weight, because you'll feel free to be your best self.

Billie is an artist in her early 50s. She came to therapy to try and improve her low self-esteem. Her mother had neglected her terribly, and she grew up feeling unlovable and undeserving of happiness. She had a compulsive eating problem, and being overweight made her feel that much more worthless. In therapy, the initial focus of healing was for her to see the truth about her past: to recognize that the way she'd been brought up was a reflection of her mother's inability to love rather than Billie's inadequacy. Once she had this realization, the work has been to get her to love and accept herself as she is, in order that positive change might happen with regard to her eating behavior and in her life.

Like Billie, if you've been overweight for a time, you may have a poor self-image. A vicious circle is created, where you overeat to comfort and care for yourself and then the internalized parent criticizes the child within for being overweight and your self-esteem plummets. This leads you to comfort yourself with more food. It doesn't help if you've also been taking to heart the criticism of your friends, family, or society, with regard to your weight.

The good news is that for Billie and for you, change is possible, but never in the context of self-hatred or attempting to meet impossible expectations. Self-acceptance is an essential aspect of change. When you lack self-acceptance or reject your body because you see it as "unattractive," it's the negative internalized parent who's criticizing the child within.

If a parent constantly criticizes her child's weight or continually draws attention to it, the child will often respond by holding on to the weight and might even gain more weight, out of despair or spite. It's been made abundantly clear by researchers that in order to enlist a child's cooperation, *loving encouragement* is what's needed. It is exactly the same within the psyche: no weight loss is possible in the deadlock that's created out of a parent-child war. In this internal power struggle the child will always prevail, until the adult self steps in to mediate.

The adult self can break the parent-child deadlock in a simple way. First, by taking on the aspect of the inner warrior, the adult can reject the internalized parent's cruel and false criticisms of the child within. The warrior can tell the child not to pay attention to these hurtful lies. Then the loving, nurturing adult self can soothe the hurt and angry child, praising and encouraging her so as to help overcome her hostility or despair.

The adult can be warmly supportive to the child within, saying, "I love you, whatever weight you are, but let's be healthier. We don't need to be constantly thinking about food and weight. Let's have more fun and be more productive." Weight loss is possible if the *adult* has chosen to do it for the *right reasons*. It can't be in relation to any internal or external pressure to be thin, but for the goals of good health, real fulfillment, and freedom from any obsession or compulsion regarding food, eating, and weight.

Our society is extremely critical of overweight people, and especially of overweight women. Women are expected to be attractive, as if they owe it to men and even to other women to be always pleasant to behold. When women aren't within the acceptable limits of what's an "attractive" weight, men and women alike regard these women as though they were purposefully deviating from the norm.

It's considered almost an affront to society for a woman not to conform to the expectations of how she "ought to" present herself. If she's overweight, a woman is seen as a subversive societal element, refusing to conform. Both male and female celebrities who dare to break their implicit beauty contract by gaining weight are subject to vicious attacks in the media, including having unflattering photographs displayed on the front pages of the tabloids and online for all to see. This is their punishment for going against expectations of what people in the public eye "should" weigh.

Overweight people are also considered "weak," "lazy," "self-indulgent," and even *morally suspect* because they appear to lack self-control. In reality, this group is only one among the many types of people engaged in compulsive behaviors or addictions. Other people can hide the fact that they drink, use drugs, view porn, shop, or gamble compulsively, but it's obvious to everyone that overweight people are this way because they overeat. The bodies of over-weight women demonstrate their "moral failings."

Some people can have serious addictions that are not recognized as a problem because these fall into the category of socially acceptable behaviors. These include being compulsive with work, helping others, food restricting, or exercise. These individuals may be in complete denial about their problem. Society colludes with them, encouraging them to work more, exercise more, do more for others, and continue to restrict food. These individuals are suffer-ing just as much from their obsessions and compulsive behaviors as any other addict, but they have a *free pass* in society because it's considered acceptable to be compulsive and miserable if it's "for a good cause," whereas it's unac-ceptable if it's for something as "self-indulgent" as overeating.

How, then, as an overweight person, can you come to love and accept yourself as you are? You must begin by rejecting the negative messages of the internalized parent and then let go of all external sources of shame and blame, including the media, loved ones and especially the hypercritical diet, exercise and lifestyle gurus around you. You need to recognize that being overweight has nothing to do with your value as a human being.

Loving and accepting yourself can't be based on your appearance or per-formance. Everyone starts out as an innocent infant who should, ideally, develop self-confidence and self-esteem through being loved, accepted, and protected by her parents or guardians. The biggest lie you're living with is that your value should be measured by how your parents or other adults treated you when you were growing up. According to this lie, if you weren't adequately loved or cared for, it's because there's something wrong with you.

The truth is that your value is independent of how your parents or guard-ians felt or acted toward you. Every child is lovable and special in her own right. You're lovable simply because you exist and you'll be loved by those who are able to do so.

Ideally, if biology were the only force involved in raising children, parents would by nature love their children and these children would grow up feeling lovable, valuable, and deserving of good things. Unfortunately, humans are ruled not only by our instincts but also by our minds, emotions, culture, and experiences. Any mental, emotional, or social problems a parent has will affect how he relates to his child, and in turn, what this child comes to believe about herself. Sadly, rather than biology being the driving force in child-rearing, culture and psychology have taken over. Many parents are wounded to some degree and these wounds have gotten in the way of their ability to do what would otherwise come naturally.

Fortunately, self-love is available to you, whether or not your parents or guardians gave you enough love and care. The adult part of the psyche can take over and give the child within love and nurturing today. People who were insufficiently loved or nurtured in the past can develop self-love in the present by having the adult spend time building a connection with the child within or by entering some type of therapy to get help in learning how to do so.

Human beings are instinctively wired for love. Loving feelings ensure that you'll nurture your young, be caring toward others and ultimately allow for survival of the species. Without love, people would have no problem abandoning their young and killing each other off, and humanity would die out. Self-love makes you care about yourself, but it also enables you to care about others, as it connects you to everyone through love. A lack of self-love, in contrast, causes alienation and is responsible, not just for self-destructive behavior, but for much of the hatred that people exhibit toward others today. As you look around and see the manifestations of this tragic hatefulness in the world, you'll recognize the importance of reconnecting with the child within in a loving way, for your own good and for the good of humanity.

We humans are complicated, in part, because we have two types of intelligence: an intellectual one and an emotional one, and these are often at odds. A person might be intellectually brilliant, with a high IQ, but could rate low in emotional intelligence, or EQ. The IQ is something we're born with and it remains stable throughout life unless it's damaged by a physical injury to the brain. The EQ has two components: one from nature and one from the environment. It's true that some people are born more sensitive and compassionate and some with less ability to empathize with others, but it's equally true that a person can become more or less emotionally in tune, depending on their childhood experiences.

People with a high IQ can exhibit amazing analytical and reasoning abilities, but they can't compete with high-EQ people when it comes to their ability to form meaningful attachments or to demonstrate empathy and compassion toward others. A person's history of emotional wounding must always be seen in the context of their unique character formation. Childhood wounds could potentially cause someone to be more insensitive, competitive, or self-serving. Depending on how resilient or vulnerable they were to begin with, these wounds could conceivably interfere with their ability to love.

In this way, intelligent, successful people can become parents while being inadequate to the needs of their children or even hurtful toward them. The child born to such parents doesn't grow up with the kind of affirmation that she can internalize and use as a model by which the adult self could love the child within. The good news is that, because everyone is instinctively hardwired for love, these unloved children have a chance to develop self-love later on in life.

Most of the people I encounter in my therapy practice are there because they weren't sufficiently loved or protected by their parents or guardians and were subsequently unable to develop self-love. Still, almost every one of them has been able to love others. These wounded individuals have life partners, good friends, or a beloved pet. Some have children for whom they've tried their best to care. It's evident that, although these people haven't sufficiently learned how to love themselves, their capacity for this is demonstrated by their ability to love and nurture others.

If you're struggling with a lack of self-love, there's hope. If you're able to be there for others, you can learn to be there for yourself. You just have to take that innate hardwiring for love and reroute it to the child within. This will allow you to create the type of loving adult-child connection that didn't happen between you and your parents.

A significant part of therapy consists of helping people learn how to become an empowered adult; to reject the negative self-talk of the internalized parent and begin to love the child within. The fact that someone has come for therapy indicates that there's a seed of self-love driving them to acknowledge their unhappiness and make different choices in order to have a better life.

To build self-love, you can do the visualization of meeting the child within and talk to the child in this context, or you can try another exercise. It's very helpful to have a symbolic representation of the child when you're working on loving and affirming this aspect of yourself. I recommend purchasing a doll or stuffed animal that will represent the child part of you. Having a symbolic child to hold is helpful in a number of ways: it immediately clarifies who's the adult and who's the child. It's impossible to identify as the child within when you're holding (a representation of) the child in your arms.

As soon as you pick up this symbolic child, you automatically become the adult who is giving her the love and affirmation she needs. It also makes the adult-child connection feel real when you're communicating with an actual "child." The feelings you have for her grow clear and strong over time.

It's helpful to find time every day to be with this symbolic child, holding her, talking to her, loving her, and even grieving your losses with her. You'll be surprised at how powerful the connection to the child will be and how quickly you begin to feel a deep love for her. If there's a voice in you that's saying that getting a doll or stuffed animal is "stupid," "foolish," or "a waste of time," it's the inner critic being contemptuous of your work in trying to heal. Don't forget, the critic wants to stay in control of you so it would be threatened by a strong adult-child bond. Don't let the inner critic undermine your efforts in building self-love by shaming you.

Self-love (the love the adult self has for the child within) allows for positive change, because it makes you feel entitled to have a better life. On the other hand, self-judgment, self-criticism, and especially self-hatred (the negative regard of the inner critic toward the child within) will make change impossible. *Negativity is like psychic glue,* making you hold on to every hurtful belief you've accumulated from your past.

When there's no self-acceptance, the hurt and angry child will sabotage any adult efforts to make positive changes. It's the adult's responsibility to make the child within feel loved and accepted and if you haven't, the child isn't going to feel connected to you. She won't be willing to cooperate with you, even when you're trying to do something good for yourself. This is why it's so important to build an alliance with the child. You both need to be on the same side, pursuing positive change and combating the internalized parent's negativity.

Behavioral changes are helpful but they aren't the primary way to lose weight. Any real change has to be motivated by emotional nurturing and healing. Emotional changes brought about by self-healing and self-love will create a new way of looking at yourself and food, and these will enable the weight to fall away. You'll no longer be trying to force the pounds off; you'll lose the urge to overeat to soothe your pain or compensate for what's missing in your life.

Having said this, there are still patterns of behavior that need to change and new habits to be adopted that will support the process of letting go of your overeating. Behavioral support that's focused on emotional healing and nurturing (as opposed to dieting) is helpful in creating change. Putting aside some time each day to tune in to the needs and feelings of the child within and to give her affirmation is an important part of the process. You'll also need to make a new habit of identifying and rejecting the negative self-talk when it comes along. These new habits will help silence the internalized parent and allow the child within to cooperate in making positive changes.

It's only through self-love that the child will find peace and be able to let go of the pursuit of love and healing through overeating or an alternative compulsive behavior. When the child finally feels truly loved, accepted, and protected by the adult, you'll be free to live your life without the burden of food or weight obsession and compulsive eating. At last you'll be able to pursue your goals and dreams from a place of an adult who wants to be happy, rather than a child who needs love and healing. In this way, self-love enables an adult to live fully in the present, no longer encumbered by the wounds of the past.

Self-love includes accepting your body the way it is right now. This doesn't mean being complacent about it, but simply understanding what brought your body to this point and making the conscious choice to deal with the real reasons why you overeat. Hatred of the body, like all self-hatred, halts the process of change because it activates the despair or resistance of the child within. Acceptance of your size and shape will enable change to occur and is an essential part of the process of healing the child's wounds, and your life.

If you as an adult can accept the body you're living in and reject internal or external criticisms about your weight and shape, you can then take responsibility for this body and make different choices about how you'll care for it in the future.

Self-acceptance goes hand in hand with personal responsibility. The adult takes responsibility for how and why she's become overweight, but does so with an attitude of compassion and understanding. This allows the child to cooperate with the process of healing and change. Accepting yourself doesn't mean being lenient. In fact, self-acceptance motivates you to do better, because it provides an atmosphere of support and encouragement in which the child is happy to participate.

Suzie's Story

Let me share a story about Suzie, who told me at the beginning of our work together that one morning, she looked at herself in the mirror and was shocked. She thought, "I can't believe I got this fat! Where was I when this was happening?" She had put on 80 pounds but hadn't really noticed the weight piling on. The child within was in charge of her eating, and this child was in denial of the weight gain.

Suzie's adult awareness was so far in the background that she'd been unconscious of her steadily increasing weight. Suddenly, the adult in her came to the forefront long enough to see what was happening, and it was at this point that she knew she had to make some real changes. It was also when the concept of ruthless compassion had to come into play if Suzie was to have any chance of success in her eating, weight, and life.

Ruthless Compassion

The concept of "ruthless compassion" brings together two of the main themes in my practice of psychotherapy. By ruthlessness, I mean the unrelenting pursuit of the unvarnished truth without allowing avoidance, fantasy, or denial to get in the way. It's the insistence on respect for oneself such that disrespect isn't tolerated. Conscious ruthlessness means that there is no enabling of others' bad behavior. It also means that there's no codependency and that adults take full responsibility for their choices.

Active compassion is the constructive use of compassion. It's an attitude of understanding that every choice you make has meaning and motivation. If you're unconscious of your needs, feelings, and urges, your life choices are being made automatically. Having compassion means that when you confront your choices in the light of the unvarnished truth, you needn't criticize yourself for any mistakes you might have made; you simply recognize your bad choices for what they are and choose to do things differently in the future.

Having compassion means that you understand the difference between real kindness and being an enabler and that you stop supporting others when they make bad choices (with regard to you or themselves), because you know it's not helpful. This means not depriving them of the natural consequences for their hurtful or dysfunctional behaviors, but allowing them to learn from their mistakes. True compassion is doing the right thing, even if other people don't understand, disapprove, or become angry.

In the absence of conscious awareness, every person is doomed to continually repeat his or her automatic patterns of thinking, feeling, and acting until consciousness comes in and can be used to break these patterns. Compassion shouldn't be confused with an attitude in which you don't hold yourself accountable for your actions. Rather, it means that you take full responsibility for the consequences of your choices, but with kindness toward yourself.

When you're compassionate as well as ruthlessly intolerant of disrespect, you'll no longer automatically accept the hurtful actions of others *because you understand them*. Active compassion helps you see that people do things for reasons of their own and not because of something you've done. Conscious ruthlessness enables you to see that just because you know *why* a person is doing something it doesn't make his behavior acceptable. When you no longer have to swallow this hurtful behavior, you'll no longer have to wash it down with food (or anything else).

With an attitude of ruthless compassion toward your own choices, you'll be able to see yourself honestly but without cruel self-criticism. In this way, the next time you have an opportunity to recognize a mistake and make a change in your attitude or behavior, you won't avoid dealing with it, because it won't automatically be associated with intolerable self-criticism.

In terms of weight gain, being ruthless means that the adult has to come to the forefront so that you can be completely honest with yourself about the underlying reasons for your eating habits and the fact that you're overweight. The role of the adult is to banish the inner critic and all the counterproductive self-judgment it brings. The compassionate adult part of you will understand that you've been wounded and that your overeating has nothing to do with a deficiency of character. With this new awareness, you'll be able to change.

When you become conscious of an attitude or behavior that isn't moving you in the direction of happiness or success, ruthless compassion will give you a new way of dealing with things. Rather than engaging in self-criticism, you'll be able to praise yourself for having the courage to face the truth, for example, about the way you've been eating.

If seeing the truth is accompanied by pride about having faced your issues head-on, rather than by criticism for having seen that you've been doing something "wrong," you'll be motivated to continue the process of changing for the better. Living with ruthless compassion allows you to face reality and take responsibility for your actions with no bitter taste in your mouth, and therefore no need to sweeten things with sugar.

You may think it's possible to control things, but that's an illusion. There's no control in life, only choices you can make about how to deal with the way things are. You can't control the weather, other people, or even your body, but you can always behave in ways that will maximize the possibility of success and you can respond to challenges in the most conscious, realistic adult manner possible. It doesn't work to be in denial and then get clobbered over the head when inevitably, reality must be faced. It also doesn't work to try to force things to be the way you want. Ruthless compassion will enable you to face the fact that *conscious choice* is the only viable option. It will prevent you from feeling frustrated or ashamed about not being able to control things the way the internalized parent says you "should."

For example, the internalized parent says that you should be able to control your appetite, but when the urge to overeat comes up, you find that you can't. Ruthless compassion allows you to recognize that there's a wounded child within you who's hungry for love and healing, and that controlling your appetite will only cause further feelings of deprivation. Ruthless compassion shows you that it's dealing with the child's needs, feelings, and beliefs underlying the urge to overeat that will enable you to make better choices about eating.

When someone isn't self-aware, they often react to people and situations with behavior that's unconsciously driven by the wounded child within. Becoming conscious is looking inward and recognizing your motivations, needs, and feelings. Responding consciously to what's really going on, within you and around you gives you the power to make positive changes for yourself. Ruthless compassion helps you wake up and face the truth, which will enable you to respond to situations as an empowered adult instead of reacting as a hurt or needy child.

For example, in the past, you may have reacted to stress by buying a lot of junk food and having a binge. Ruthless compassion allows you to stop before or during your shopping trip, face the truth about what you're on the verge of doing and ask yourself, "is a binge what I really need?" You could then go home and give the child within some loving attention, instead.

Without ruthless compassion, it's difficult to stop and face your actions there and then because that would give the inner critic an opportunity to condemn you for "doing something stupid." With ruthless compassion, you can feel good about having recognized that you're making the wrong choice and you then can make a better one.

Even if consciousness kicks in when you've already begun the binge, ruthless compassion will still help you. You'll see that you're always able to face and stop this behavior and turn to the thing you really need right now. This choice is preferable to staying unconscious and continuing the binge out of the fear that seeing the truth will shame you.

The good news is that the more you practice becoming aware of your behavior and responding to yourself with compassion, the sooner you'll be able to wake up and see what you're doing. This is how ruthless compassion will allow you to change your behavior from an automatic act of compensatory overeating to a conscious response to your true needs.

The child within is entirely self-focused and the natural narcissism of this stage in life creates a lot of suffering if it's overrepresented in your adult life. If you carry this self-centeredness into adulthood, you won't be able to keep from taking everything personally and frequently becoming hurt or angry as a result. Being an adult is seeing that the things happening around you and to you are sometimes due to choices you've made and sometimes completely unassociated with you.

The wounded child within is a true narcissist, barely capable of empathy and insensitive to the needs or suffering of others. No matter how much she hurts others or herself in her wrong-headed search for happiness and healing, she won't stop. This is due to her pathological hope and a lack of personal responsibility. She'll take and take from the world, and have nothing to offer in return. She's the true exploiter of all the resources available to her, not because she's immoral but because she's amoral—unable to appreciate the consequences of her choices.

The true adult attitude is an attitude of compassion to all. Being a fully fledged adult is about moving from being a voracious consumer to being someone who makes a contribution. Children are naturally selfish, needy, and greedy but adults are capable of generosity and altruism. As an adult, you can recognize that you're connected to the whole world and responsible for the part you play in it. You care about yourself and about those around you. If you've erred, it's up to you to make amends. This is ruthless compassion in action.

We belong to each other and to the earth, and can't continue to be parasites on it and in our relationships if we want there to be a world in the future. A child-centered attitude of endlessly consuming in order to compensate for what's missing inside only perpetuates more consumption, because nothing external ever satisfies. We'll eventually destroy all our relationships and deplete all the resources on earth if we allow this childlike attitude to prevail.

Healing the wounds that drive compulsion and addiction will allow you to shift your motivation from child-centered voraciousness to a compassionate, empowered adult desire to share, and will enable you to pursue the things that will bring real happiness.

A wounded child can't let go of anything because she has no tolerance for loss. As an adult, you can understand that it's natural for things to come and go. In terms of overeating, it means that you don't have to eat everything in front of you at this very minute, because you trust that there will always be more food. The child panics from an attitude of scarcity, believing that she needs to have more immediately to fill her need, but the adult knows that there's more down the road. At dinners and parties, the child-driven individual eats as though there's no tomorrow. But an adult is able to eat with moderation, knowing that food isn't going to heal her wounds or bring her love, and that there will always be more of it.

With an attitude of ruthless compassion, you can see the world for what it truly is, recognizing when people have been cruel or have broken the social contract of kindness, caring, and personal responsibility. The ruthlessly compassionate adult doesn't need to be in denial about the capacity for cruelty in others because she's strong enough to face the truth. Conscious ruthlessness allows you to recognize that human beings are capable of anything, from acts of the highest altruism to the lowest depths of depravity. Someone lacking ruthless compassion may feel sympathy for an oppressor, wanting only to see the wounded child within them and ignoring the fact that they're really destructive and responsible for the harm they've caused.

Practicing ruthless compassion is being respectful toward yourself and others. It's about understanding that depriving another person of the natural consequences of his actions is disrespectful, as it enables him to persist in his destructive behavior and deprives him of the opportunity to change. An adult with ruthless compassion doesn't collude with anyone who's cruel or hurtful, and doesn't protect him from the outcomes of his choices.

By seeing the truth about others, you'll be safer in the world. When you live in reality, as opposed to child-like idealism, you're no longer compelled to deny that others can be harmful or destructive. You'll stop thinking, "I can't believe that this person could be so cruel," or even, "I refuse to believe that this person is capable of having done such a terrible thing," or worse, yet, "I understand why this person was hurtful, so that makes it acceptable." Instead, as a ruthlessly compassionate person, you'll face the truth about everyone with whom you interact. You needn't feel sorry for a person who's disrespectful toward you, seeing only the wounded child within them. You'll know that it's the adult who's ultimately responsible for their behavior.

Although it might not come naturally or easily, it's definitely possible for everyone to develop ruthless compassion. This way of being is the way of love, change, and truth. By love, I mean a sense of interconnectedness and interdependence among all living things. By change, I mean a shaking up of the status quo, of the beliefs you're living with today that promote avoidance and denial, materialism, and consumerism, as opposed to consciousness, responsibility, caring, and sharing. And by truth, I mean the willingness to be grounded in reality and use your powers of observation to see what's really happening in front of you, as opposed to believing what you want to believe, based on false hope and wishful thinking.

By practicing ruthless compassion, you'll see that everything is connected; every choice you make has consequences that affect you and the world. You don't act in vacuum, and knowing this moves you to take responsibility for your part in the grand scheme of things. By allowing yourself to experience interconnectedness and interdependence, you'll be able to develop ruthless compassion. Ultimately, ruthless compassion is about questioning things, not with cynicism but with a sincere desire to get at the truth. It comes from the practical, rational adult part of the psyche—one that's sadly deficient in many people today.

Many of us behave like children or adolescents much of the time because we're carrying unhealed wounds and unmet needs from the past that keep the child-mind in the forefront of the psyche. We can choose to deal with our "unfinished business" and wake up, grow up and become accountable for our actions. Acting as an adult and taking responsibility for yourself requires tolerating the fact that some of your needs won't be met right away, but you'll soon discover that it's worth it for the sake of true, long-term fulfillment. The child within abhors deferred gratification because she believes that she won't survive unless she gets what she wants immediately.

The adult, on the other hand, has learned from experience that sometimes, something that's hard-won is that which she can most savor, and that grabbing the first thing she sees often has negative consequences. The adult understands that working and waiting for the right thing lead to happiness and fulfillment, whereas acting without thinking creates suffering.

The child within is incapable of taking responsibility for her choices, and blames others for what she's done or what's happened to her. "He made me do it!" cries the little one after she's knocked over the lamp. As I said before, in adults this is victim consciousness. We believe that if our lives are going badly, it's not because we've made the wrong choices, but because we've been persecuted or led astray. Unfortunately, when you see yourself as a victim, you've given up the power to improve your life. You're dependent on others to rescue you from the situations in which you find yourself and you're at the mercy of these rescuers.

The adult who's accountable doesn't blame others for the choices she's made. The adult's compassionate attitude enables her to face her own mistakes and make better choices in the future. This enables her to have a better life with less suffering, and can alleviate the need for overeating or any other addiction as the way to deal with her pain.

Becoming a fully fledged adult will happen when you begin taking better care of the child within and addressing the inner conflict between child and parent parts of the psyche. Making the choice to grow up supports the development of ruthless compassion, and developing ruthless compassion helps you become an adult.

Some of us today are susceptible to the lies we're told about the nature of people and things, because these lies seemingly let us off the hook for the problems in our life. The child within is happy to avoid the truth, because she doesn't believe she can tolerate it and she's convinced that she's powerless to change anything. The perpetrators of the lies are promoting their own agendas by deceiving the public with disinformation and false promises.

I'll give you an example: A diet program misinforms when it promises that you can lose weight and keep it off with minimal time and effort. This lie is evident in every diet ad on TV or in print, where if you look closely, you'll see the tiny proviso at the bottom of the picture of a newly svelte woman that reads, "Results not typical." There is also no mention of how hard this woman actually worked to lose the weight or long she's been able to keep the weight off. Sadly, some of us so desperately want to believe that we can lose weight permanently on the diet being promoted that we ignore the obvious deception and choose to believe, instead, that we'll be just like this so-called success story.

The people pictured in diet ads don't represent a successful diet or indicate that the majority of us can succeed, long-term, with the diet being advertised. These people either have won the battle of willpower for the moment, or they've lost weight for reasons other than the diet, perhaps because they were emotionally ready to let go of their compulsive eating. The program takes credit when someone loses weight and blames it on the dieter if they haven't. In fact, those whose good results are "not typical" are a very tiny minority of the hundreds of thousands of people each year who've gone on diets in the false hope of losing weight.

You can naively continue to believe the lies you're being told or you can begin to question the diet industry. "Show us the statistics," you could say to a diet program you're considering, "what are the long-term success rates of your plan, and what's really involved in someone losing the weight and keeping it off?" In this way, you can bring ruthless compassion to your investigation of the diet industry and can see it for the what it truly is, which would then lead you to seek more viable solutions to your problems of overeating and being overweight.

The attitude of ruthless compassion means having a healthy sense of skepticism. Rather than simply believing what you're told because it pleases the child within who's attracted to quick and easy solutions, you have another option. You can ask yourself, "How does this company benefit by promoting their diet?" and "What's in it for me if I go on the diet? Is it safe? Will I be wasting my time and money? Will I be jeopardizing my health if the diet fails and my weight goes up and down?" Being overly credulous is a child-like attitude that allows us to be easily deceived or exploited. By developing an attitude of healthy skepticism, you'll be on your way to freedom from the lies that profit others but imprison you in fruitless pursuits.

Ruthless compassion is associated with the understanding that we can't control the way things are. What we have, instead, is the power of conscious choice. You may be someone who overeats because you feel out of control in your life. Eating initially soothes your anxious, hurt, or lonely feelings. After you've had your binge, however, you feel even more out of control than before. The internalized parent then tries to impose control on the child within, which makes her react with despair or anger and further overeating. The way to break this vicious circle is to understand that letting go of compulsive eating is not a matter of finally "being in control."

If you feel out of control in your life, you must realize that this is because the child within is in charge, and your adult self is not. The internalized parent's attempts at controlling the child within will only backfire. When the adult takes over as the primary identity, you'll be able to let go of the notion of "control" and make conscious, empowered choices as opposed to impulsive, reactive, counterproductive ones. This will cause you to have fewer negative consequences and will make you feel more in charge of yourself.

The development of ruthless compassion requires conscious attention and a certain amount of discipline. You must want to change your pattern of self-criticism and feeling helpless or overwhelmed. You'll need to work at overcoming old, entrenched beliefs about yourself, others, and the world and instead start facing the truth about these things. This may seem like a daunting task, but the payoff is enormous. Living with ruthless compassion will improve your life on every level, and it will make addiction a thing of the past.

FACING, GRIEVING, AND LETTING GO

The healing process for overeating and other addictions will take some time and energy, but will absolutely yield results. Even though the process may take several months, you'll start to feel better right away and you'll see positive changes quite quickly. As I talked about earlier, the process begins with you *facing the truth* about your childhood.

It's essential to be honest with yourself about what you missed out on as a child, and what bad things may have happened to you. It may be painful to see the truth in such a clear light but unless you know the full extent of your emotional wound, you won't be able to heal every aspect of it. Information is power and the more you know about your past, the more power you have to heal it.

The next part of the healing process, as I said previously, is *grieving your losses,* the loss of what you needed as a child and the loss of innocence caused by exploitation or abuse. The grieving process takes time, as any does type of normal grieving, but at the end of it you should be left with a sense of freedom and inner peace.

ACTIVE GRIEVING

Here's an exercise for grieving the losses of your past: hold the doll or stuffed animal that you use as the symbolic representation of the child within. Relax, and let your mind be open to any feelings or memories that may come up in relation to the past.

Talk to the child within, and begin by acknowledging that she's been hurt. Tell her you're so sorry that bad things happened to her or that her needs weren't met, and that you're here now to love her and protect her from harm. Hold her close and feel a sense of deep compassion for the suffering she's experienced.

Surprising memories might come up and new feelings might arise within you. You may need to do this exercise a few times before the child within feels safe enough to let her memories and feelings become conscious to you. If something does come up, just receive it without trying to analyze it. Let yourself be moved and if tears come, let them flow. (After the exercise is over, you might want to think about what came up for you and try to make sense of it then. You can do this on your own or with a therapist. The important thing is that the active grieving exercise should be a time to remember and have your feelings, rather than trying to figure things out.)

Of course, if tears begin to flow, it's you who'll be crying, but you'll experience it as the child within shedding her tears. As you cry, hug the child within, giving her love and support. She'll cry for as long as she needs, and when you're done you should feel a deep sense of relief.

Perhaps, in one of these active grieving exercises, you were able to access a memory that had been buried since childhood. The more time you spend with the child within, the more she'll trust you and allow previously unconscious material to be available to your conscious awareness.

Retrieving these buried memories and experiencing the associated emotions will give you an opportunity to fully grieve all your hurts and losses. In the process, you might discover some upsetting information that's been repressed until now. If anything is coming up that you're uncomfortable dealing with on your own, this would be a good time to contact a psychotherapist, so that you can address this information with someone experienced in helping.

The final part of the process of healing is when you're able to *let go of the past* and live fully in the present. This happens naturally as the end point of the grieving process. When you let go of the past, the child within is no longer compelled to pursue dysfunctional methods to fix it or get other people to compensate for it. Your actions will no longer be geared toward resolving your childhood wounds, but instead will be focused on creating a good life for yourself in the present.

There's no way to ever make up for what you missed out on as a child, and no way to take away the bad things that happened to you. By grieving your losses, however, you'll finally be able to let go of the hurt, pain, and longing for healing. You can't go back and rewrite the script of your childhood, but the child within can finally be soothed and comforted in a meaningful way and can finally receive the love and nurturing she's always needed, from you the adult. It's empowering to know that *you are all you need for your healing*. No one and nothing else is necessary. In fact, it's counterproductive to attempt to get anyone else involved in this process other than a therapist, whose job is not to heal you but to facilitate your process of change.

Many of my patients thought it would help them heal if they were to confront their parents with complaints about their childhood. Many believed that if their parents were to accept responsibility for having hurt or disappointed them, this would enable them to heal. A few of my patients had tried this before beginning their therapy process with me. Rather than bringing them healing, these attempts at confrontation either made no difference in their lives or created terrible conflicts in which the parents denied that anything bad had ever happened, said that my patient was imagining things, or even accused my patient of trying to destroy the family with their lies.

I don't recommend that you look to your parents or guardians to help with your healing. First of all, it puts the healing process in the hands of other people, and puts you in the same helpless position you were in as a child, hoping and waiting for your parents to come through for you. If your parents refuse to acknowledge what really happened and say that you're remembering incorrectly, exaggerating, or trying to make trouble, it will only reinforce your wounds.

If your parents let you down while you were growing up, why would you believe that they'd come through for you now? If they were inadequate parents back then, they aren't likely to take responsibility for their past mistakes today. Waiting for your parents to acknowledge your wounds and make up for their failings puts your healing in the hands of the people who hurt you in the first place. This attempt at confrontation comes out of the pathological hope of the child within that she can, once and for all, get the love and healing from them that she's always longed for.

Even if your parents were basically loving and caring and the wounds you developed while growing up were due to their being wounded themselves, receiving an acknowledgment or an apology from them still can't heal your wounds. Each of my patients has had to learn this lesson: no other person can heal your wounds, even if he caused the wounds in the first place. Once you've been wounded, your wound is your own possession and your own responsibility and no matter how well-intentioned another person is, he can't take over your healing.

Your parents might have caused you to be wounded in the past, but today, the wounds are yours alone to heal. If you insist on trying to get others to heal these wounds for you, your focus will be in the wrong place, your power will be in others' hands and you'll never heal. Every adult must take responsibility for herself, which in part means letting go of trying to get the people who hurt you to heal you.

VISUALIZATION 3: COMBATING THE INNER OPPONENT

In healing the wounds of childhood, it's essential to eliminate, as much as possible, the negative voice of the internalized parent. As I said earlier, this voice can be in the form of the inner critic, inner opponent, or even inner killer. In whatever form, it oppresses and paralyzes the child within and prevents you from being happy and fulfilled in your adult life.

Sitting quietly on a comfortable, straight-backed chair in a private room where you won't be disturbed, plant your feet on the ground, relax your body and bring your attention to your breathing. Allow the air to enter all the way down into your belly, without effort, and then allow the air to flow out from your belly with the same ease. Gently, easily, you're inhaling and exhaling and as you breathe, you feel at peace.

Picture yourself back in your small, cozy room. Look around and see everything in its place. You're sitting in the beautiful, comfortable chair and in front of you is the small, child-sized door. Hanging on the wall facing you, to your right, is a large, full-length mirror in an ornate gilded frame. High in the wall to the left of the door is a small, round window and below it against the wall facing you stand three tall earthenware urns.

Now bring your attention to the door in front of you. It opens, and once again, coming through it is the child within. Notice if she's changed since the last time you saw her. Is she younger or older? Is she happy to see you? Welcome her and bring her up onto the chair with you. Get in touch with what it feels to be with this child again and notice how she feels, sitting with you in the chair.

Next, bring your attention to the large mirror on the wall. As you look at it, the glass begins to fog up and then the fog begins to swirl. It swirls and swirls, and then retreats to the edges of the mirror, leaving only the empty frame. Within the frame, you see a long tunnel extending way back. From far in the distance, you see a being approaching you. It's your inner warrior. Notice if it's the same warrior you met in the previous visualization or a different one. Know that whatever manifestation it takes, it's still your inner warrior, here to protect and defend you. How do you feel, seeing the warrior here today? How is the child reacting?

The warrior comes to the edge of the frame, and then steps out and comes to stand in front of you and bows. You greet your warrior and thank it for coming to be with you. Then, the warrior takes its place in front of you, facing the small window high in the wall to the left of the door. You see something coming into the room through this window. It's a smoky, greasy apparition: your inner opponent. It floats down to face the inner warrior and may take on a more physical shape, or remain in its greasy, smoky form.

Immediately, the warrior is upon it, attacking this opponent with all its weapons, pulverizing it until nothing remains but a gooey mess. The warrior then scoops up all the remnants of the vanquished opponent and brings them to the urns.

These are magical urns, in which a fierce fire lights up at the bottom when something is put into them. The warrior dumps the remains of the opponent into one or more of the urns, and these remains are instantly incinerated and turned into smoke and ashes that float up and out through the window, to fertilize the fields beyond.

When the warrior has completed this task, it comes and stands in front of you and the child again. Thank your inner warrior for coming here today to combat and defeat the inner opponent, and listen to what the warrior might have to say to you. Notice what the child is feeling at this time, and if she has anything to say to the warrior.

Now, the warrior comes to stand behind you. Feel the warrior turn into a column of energy and light, lining up with your spine. Feel this column of energy and light merging with your spinal column. Notice that you're sitting up straighter in your chair, as the warrior energy fills your spine. Feel the power of the warrior in your spine, and know that with this energy within you, you're invincible.

With the warrior energy in your spine, hold the child to your heart. As you do so, she begins to shimmer and glisten and becomes transparent. Press the child into your heart and then feel her there, this being of love, filling your heart.

Take a moment to feel the warrior in your spine and the child in your heart. Remember what the warrior did for you today and know that you can call upon your inner warrior any time you need this fierce being to protect or defend you. Know that your warrior is more powerful than any opponent, and that nothing the opponent intends for you need come to pass if you bring the warrior to bear against it.

After a few moments, it's time to go back to the present, but carry this memory of the powerful warrior with you, as well as the sense of what the inner opponent felt like. Know that having seen this opponent and conquered it, you'll be ready the next time it emerges to recognize and defeat it.

I'd like to make a comment about the violence in this visualization. Remember that no one is being hurt by this exercise. Some people object to the violent aspects of it, but I'm not recommending taking violent action in the world; just destroying the inner opponent in the exercise. Think about it: what would you do if you had a terrible infection, or cancer? We undergo powerful treatments for these conditions that are meant to eradicate disease-causing organisms or tumors from our bodies. I see the inner opponent as equivalent to a virulent pathogen or a malignant tumor. We need to work hard at destroying it because it's interfering with our happiness and success. Allowing the inner warrior to completely defeat the inner opponent will show you that you're more powerful than this murderous psychic entity.

6

A NEW YOU EMERGING:
LETTING GO OF YOUR OLD IDENTITY

We hold beliefs without even realizing it, and our actions can contradict our conscious notions of what we believe. An example of this is a patient of mine named Karla, who seemed to be motivated in therapy and kept telling me that she was willing to do whatever it took to make changes in her weight and her life. Despite this, she never took any positive steps and there were no changes. She believed that she wanted to lose weight, but something was stopping her.

On further investigation, the adult Karla did want to change, but the child within was holding on to the belief that change was impossible. The internalized parent had been telling the child that she would forever be a "fat girl" and could never lose the weight. There was an inner conflict going on between the adult who wanted to be healthy and free of the compulsion to overeat, and the child who was convinced (by the internalized parent) that she couldn't. Until Karla was able to get in touch with these deeper child-held beliefs to see how they were being reinforced by the internalized parent, no change was possible for her.

If you're going through life convinced that you're meant to be a "fat person," this belief will prevent you from becoming thin. Letting go of the overweight identity requires the same components as any other process of change. First and foremost, any change calls for an investment of time. Our society values rapid results, but as I said before, many important things take time. When you're rushing around, preoccupied with all the minutiae of your daily life, there's no time for much-needed feeling or reflection. Change requires self-awareness. You need to slow down and take the time to get to know yourself and what you want in your life.

We're attached to our identity because of unconscious beliefs and because of the comfort of habit. What's familiar always seems better than what's different, even if the new way of being seems like it might be preferable. We cleave to the familiar out of a primal fear of the unknown, which goes right back to the infant confronting a strange new world where everything that's different seems dangerous.

The child within has great difficulty changing, but it's not just her fault. The internalized parent is rigidly attached to the status quo and strongly resists change. The parent wants things to remain unchanged for fear that it would lose its power and influence within the psyche. If you begin to change, the internalized parent sees this as a threat. The parent tells the child within that change isn't possible for her and the child believes the lie.

For this reason, you'll need to bring the adult into the forefront if you want to begin letting go of the old and embracing the new. An empowered adult doesn't believe the parental lies about how identity is immutable and change is impossible. The warrior within sees the internalized parent as the enemy of the self, and can banish its influence from the psyche.

The adult has to reassure the child that change is safe because the adult will be there to deal with whatever new experiences come with change. *Self-trust* is another crucial ingredient for change. The anxiety (the child within) you might feel about anything new or different in yourself or your life will be offset by the confidence the child feels toward the adult self. If the adult has demonstrated her competence, resilience, and resourcefulness to the child within, change won't be so frightening. You can trust yourself to cope successfully with anything new that happens in your body, your identity, and your life.

If you haven't had adequate parents, you won't have developed good self-trust because you were supposed to learn this by trusting the parents who protected and defended you and took care of you, no matter what. With inadequate or hurtful parents, the child interpreted any neglect or abandonment as a message from them that she didn't deserve to be taken care of, and also, that adults can't be trusted.

As an adult, you can begin to develop self-trust by acknowledging all of the ways that you're capable and competent and all of the ways that you're able to take care of the child within. Self-trust grows when you remember all the times that you stood up against negative internal or external messages and all the times you reassured the child within that she'd be okay. With self-trust, change is a positive step forward rather than a terrifying notion.

Empowerment is an important element as well, in being able to change your identity. If you feel strong within yourself, you'll be capable of dealing with change. Unfortunately, if you were made to feel helpless from parental abuse or neglect or because you had insecure parents who modeled fearfulness to you, you'll have internalized this anxiety and helplessness and it will have been translated into the belief that as an adult, you're incapable of change.

This belief can become a paralyzing influence on you. In order to overcome what's known as "learned helplessness," you'll need to recognize that even though you were powerless as a child, you now have access to an inner warrior who's strong enough to deal with anything frightening that might arise during the process of change and with any obstacles to change you may encounter.

Letting go of an old identity is also about letting go of the superficial way that you look at yourself. You must begin to realize that you're not simply a bundle of attributes or a label based on your appearance, values, race, religion, or class. It's easy to get so stuck on these attributes that you find yourself saying, "I'm the kind of person who always . . .," or "I personally would never . . .," or "I'm someone who couldn't possibly. . . ."

It's easy to start believing that who you are is a fixed and permanent state, rather than a flowing, changing set of traits. Yes, some things about you won't change. We're all born with innate character traits, but this doesn't mean that you can't let go of any dysfunctional attitudes, beliefs, or behaviors you might have adopted in response to childhood (or even adult-life) events. Your innate personality type is a permanent part of you, as is your IQ, body structure, and eye color. There are many acquired aspects to each personality, however, and these can change and develop over the years.

You can learn new skills and become adept at any number of things; you can gain wisdom, knowledge, and understanding. You can change your religion, your politics, and your point of view. Things can happen in your life that will change how you see yourself and the world as long as you're not so rigid that you won't let yourself be affected by these experiences. Change can also happen because you become ill or disabled in some way. You could lose a body part due to an accident or disease. Any of these things could alter who you are to some extent, but your fundamental character will remain unchanged.

Weight is not a permanent character trait. It's one attribute that can potentially fluctuate a great deal during a person's life. You could start out heavy and then lose the weight and spend the rest of your life thin, or vice versa. You could gain and lose hundreds of pounds over a lifetime. People also change their lifestyle, career choice, or sexual orientation. Liberals can become conservatives and stock brokers can go "back to the land." Carnivores can become vegans and ballerinas can obtain MBAs. Finally, if you grow old, your body and mind will change with the process of aging.

There are definitely some things about you that will remain more-or-less constant throughout life and a lot about you that will change over time. *Identity is more of a blueprint than the finished building.* It's the bones of who you are and not the flesh. Being overly attached to a particular "identity" is a sign of mental rigidity. The truth is that you exist, whether or not you're consciously aware of your identity, and you'll always be yourself, even if this "identity" changes dramatically.

If you lose 50 pounds, your superficial identity might change from being a heavy person to a thin one, but who you are remains the same. The real question is, "how rigid do you want to be in terms of how you see yourself?" The more attached you are to one fixed identity, the fewer options you have to become happier, healthier, and free from the suffering caused by dysfunctional beliefs and behaviors.

Change is inevitable. It's the one guarantee in life. The real question is, "who's going to be in charge of how you change?" You have the freedom and the power to decide whether you want to change something in your life, when to do it, and how you'll go about it. It's really up to you. In terms of letting go of the identity of a fat person and embracing that of a thin one, it's easier than you might think.

When Others Hold on to Your Old Identity

My patient Joanne, a biologist, recounted a story from years ago when she'd been trying to quit drinking. At the time she couldn't understand why her husband kept bringing home bottles of fine wine. When she ignored these bottles, demonstrating her earnestness about no longer using alcohol, her husband upped the ante. He began to drink wine in front of her most evenings, encouraging her to accompany him in this activity. He even went so far as to subtly threaten to leave her, telling her she was abandoning him when she refused to drink with him.

He was deeply invested in maintaining the status quo because he strongly, and correctly, suspected that if she became sober, she'd realize what a bad husband he was. Ultimately, despite her husband's attempts at sabotage, Joanne never resumed her drinking. Not long after this, she did leave the marriage, and she's been happy and sober ever since.

As I discussed in the section on the outer opponents in life, I've encountered more than one patient whose supposedly close friend or loving partner tried to undermine their attempts to lose weight. These people did their best to keep my patients overeating and overweight. In therapy, my patients learned an important truth: *the people who love you will want the best for you.* They won't hold you back out of fear of change. My patients learned that those who sabotage your attempts to be happier or healthier aren't your real friends and you don't owe them any loyalty.

Some people, like Joanne's husband, are afraid that if you change for the better, you might see them as no longer desirable and won't want to be their friend or partner anymore. Some people are insecure and don't believe that you love them for who they are, but that you're settling for what you can get in the moment. They fear that if you change for the better, you might drop them and "upgrade for a better model." In genuine relationships based on real intimacy and trust, a bit of reassurance should put the fears of your insecure friends or partner to rest.

In some relationships, however, your friend or your partner may have chosen you because they've noticed some particular vulnerability on your part. Maybe you have low self-esteem, a lack of confidence, or a problem with overeating. These people are taking advantage of what they perceive as a weakness in you so that they can be in the "one-up" position in the relationship. They need to feel like they're better than you and believe that if you become stronger and healthier, they'll lose their superior status.

Those who choose to be in a relationship with you specifically because you're struggling with issues such as self-esteem or weight will do everything they can to keep you from getting the help you need because it serves their purposes to keep you in the one-down position. They need to feel superior, to have the upper hand, and they'll undermine your chances for growth and healing while simultaneously claiming to be the only one who loves you as you are.

Those who are rigidly attached to your overweight or insecure identity are the "outer opponents" in your life. They're not going to allow you to build self-esteem or lose weight. If you can't get them to see what they're doing and how it's hurting you, the only choice for you will be to walk away. If you maintain relationships with people like this, you'll be dealing with a double dose of negativity toward the child within—from both inner and outer opponents.

Thinking as a Thin Person Instead of a Fat Person

In order to become a thin person, first it's necessary that you think like one. If you think like a fat person, you'll never be able to let go of the weight. Let me explain: Thinking like a thin person has less to do with your weight and more to do with your mindset. A person who's thin can begin to think like a fat person, and a heavy person can begin to think like a thin person. In fact, it's changing your thinking that leads to changes in your body, for better or worse.

In general, someone who's always been thin will think like a thin person, but if you've been overweight for a long time, you'll begin thinking like a fat person. At some point when you were a child, an adolescent or an adult, your relationship with food changed and it became a charged substance. At this point, you began to think like a fat person.

I'll give you an example: A thin-thinking person doesn't think about food all the time. She spends her days attending to the things that need to get done, including feeding herself and her family, but she doesn't focus on food any more than she focuses on her family, her finances, her job, or her leisure activities. She doesn't have conflicting emotions or obsessions about food.

Food, to a thin person, is enjoyable fuel, but not the center of her existence. Instead of being preoccupied with food, she's able to bring her attention and energy to creating the best life she can for herself and her loved ones. A thin person isn't constantly thinking about her weight. She thinks, instead, about all the important and interesting people and things in her life, her goals, and her plans. She's free of disordered habits of thinking and eating.

If you've lost weight and are now thin, but you spend your days obsessing about food or weight, then you're still thinking like a fat person. Your obsession with food and weight means that you're suffering from disordered eating. You're at high risk of regaining your weight or of taking extreme measures to keep the weight off, such as going on dangerous diets, purging, or overexercising.

If you've become thin but are still preoccupied with food, eating, and weight, you won't be happy. You'll be as miserably obsessed with food and weight as when you were heavy. In fact, you may be putting your health at risk in order to remain thin. To be healthy and truly free of addiction, you'll need to stop thinking like a fat person.

A thin-thinking woman doesn't feel at risk of succumbing to temptation. Food isn't equated with something "sinful," and eating the occasional treat isn't seen as "being bad." A thin-thinking woman is comfortable in her body. She won't be constantly obsessed with the need to change something about it. Rather than dwelling on her physical imperfections, a woman who thinks like a thin person will accept and enjoy her body while maintaining a good level of health and fitness.

A thin-thinking person sees food through adult eyes, making meal choices primarily for the purposes of good nutrition. A fat-thinking person sees food through the eyes of either the internalized parent or the child within. When you think like a thin person, you don't see food as having a moral value. Foods aren't "good" or "bad." Eating isn't about "behaving" or "being naughty." Thin-thinking people aren't caught up in a parent-child conflict, so they don't overeat in defiance or despair in reaction to parental pressure to be thin.

Thin-thinking people see food for what it is and enjoy it without overvaluing it. Fat-thinking people have a love-hate relationship with food; food is heaven and hell, ecstasy and agony, lover and demon. The child within sees food as all good, and the internalized parent sees it as potentially evil.

There's a similar difference between an alcoholic and a social drinker. The social drinker will have an occasional drink, but then won't think about drinking until the next social event comes along. The alcoholic will have a drink, but then won't be able to stop thinking about the next drink because the child within sees alcohol as the answer to her problems. Like a social drinker in relation to alcohol, a thin-thinking person isn't obsessive with respect to food.

Those who see addiction as an incurable "disease" believe that the addict must fight a daily battle to stay on the side of sobriety, but it's not inevitable that someone who thinks like a fat person must be obsessed with food, weight, and dieting forever. She isn't doomed to spend the rest of her life battling against her addiction. There's a way to achieve real freedom from alcohol, compulsive eating, or any other addiction. You don't have to be constantly thinking about food, tormented about whether to resist the urge to overeat or give in to your cravings.

You don't have to live your life feeling guilty because you're always tempted to eat the "wrong" foods when you know you should be eating the "right" foods. You can let go of the obsessive thinking about food and weight that's the hallmark of thinking like a fat person and begin thinking like a thin person. It's about taking the charge off food and eating, rather than anything to do with how much you weigh. In fact, to lose weight, you must first change your thinking. When food and eating are no longer such charged subjects, your behavior will change and the weight will begin to come off.

A thin-thinking person isn't caught up in parental self-judgment or perfectionism about food. She's able to enjoy the occasional indulgence without giving herself a psychological whipping. She's a reasonable adult around her food choices and doesn't allow the inner critic to attack the child within if she craves or eats something fattening or unhealthy on occasion.

If you're a strong adult, you'll be able to heal and nurture the child within and banish the inner opponent. This will make it possible for you to think like a thin person and to break the spell that food once had over you. Healing your wounds and taking real care of the child will enable food to lose its charge and become "neutralized," as opposed to something you obsess over. As an adult, you'll be free to make the types of responsible choices about food and eating that most lovingly support your physical well-being.

CORA'S STORY

One of my patients several years ago made a strong impression on me because her situation was so unusual. Cora was a young artist who spent hours and hours in her studio painting. She admitted to me that she "got high" doing art, and that during the times she wasn't paining, she experienced something similar to withdrawal symptoms. She was so hooked on this activity that she let her relationships and many other aspects of her life fall by the wayside.

Cora is an example of a personality type that's more at risk for overeating and for addiction in general: this is the "ecstatic" personality that has been described in various writings on addiction. This personality type desires ecstatic or "peak" experiences and strongly craves the feeling of being in an altered or euphoric state. People like this tend to have more trouble with addiction than the rest of the population because of how they experience these highs. Recent scientific findings indicate that this might be, in part, because their brain doesn't register them as powerfully as the average person. The brain has something called a "reward pathway," in which the neurotransmitter dopamine is involved in mediating pleasure responses and is implicated in addictive behavior.

Writing in a *New York Times* article,[1] David J. Linden, a professor of neuroscience at Johns Hopkins University School of Medicine explains that some individuals are born with a gene that causes decreased dopamine release in response to pleasurable activities, and that they enjoy these pleasurable activities less as a result, which in turn leads to an increase in pleasure-seeking and novelty-seeking behaviors.

According to Steven E. Hyman of the National Institute of Mental Health, in a paper titled, "The Addicted Brain,"[2] repeated drug use reduces the production of dopamine in the reward pathway, which causes a blunted experience of pleasure. Some recent research suggests that this is the case for other addicts, as well. Whatever is happening in the brains of these individuals, they feel a much greater need to engage in pleasure-seeking, stimulating activities.

Ecstatic personalities make up a large percentage of the populations in rehab centers and weight-loss clinics. Many artists, actors, musicians, and athletes are novelty-seeking ecstatic types, and this is, in part, what makes them able to express their talents so well. It's also, unfortunately, what gets them into trouble, like the actor addicted to cocaine, the athlete hooked on gambling, or the extremely overweight singer. Not every overeater or addict is an ecstatic type, and not every person with an ecstatic personality is struggling with addiction, but many are. If you have such a personality, how can you restrain your addictive impulses while remaining true to your nature?

BALANCE AND GROUNDING

Like with every personality type, the ecstatic personality has its positive and negative aspects: on the positive side, such a person can be artistic, open-minded, and willing to take risks. This explains why so many creative individuals have this personality type. On the negative side, people with ecstatic personalities can be self-absorbed, impulsive, and even self-destructive as they search for the next "high." They can also be fanatical or irrational as they relentlessly pursue thrills over responsibility. Examples of this can be found in members of religious cults, political extremists, or extreme athletes. A person who has just a few of these traits could be artistic and charismatic, but also have a tendency to overindulge in pleasurable activities like eating, drinking, or socializing.

Since at this point in time we're unable to affect the neurobiology of pleasure-seeking behavior, the answer to how to maintain the positive aspects of this type of personality while not succumbing to the negatives must be psychological. In fact, it lies in two basic principles: *balance and grounding.* It's important to recognize the value of the peak experience while knowing that it must exist in balance with the more mundane life experiences. The "highs" in life give great pleasure and joy in the same way sugar, salt, or pepper enhance the flavor of food. In the same way that too much intense seasoning is bad for you, there has to be a balance of highs and more ordinary states so that you can have a stable and healthy existence.

Grounding is the process of calming yourself down, relaxing, and literally feeling the ground beneath your feet. This is essential in helping anyone with ecstatic traits maintain a stable existence. Grounding helps you come "down to earth." Someone who loves to fly high needs this the most. The ecstatic personality craves what are known as "transcendent" experiences or those that make you feel like you're going beyond mundane reality. The problem with this is that if you're not spending enough time in reality, you won't be dealing with your problems in a realistic way and are probably creating all sorts of consequences in the meantime. Grounding allows you to be joyful and creative, while avoiding the accumulation of consequences.

GROUNDING EXERCISES

One simple grounding exercise is to sit in a straight-backed chair and remove your shoes. Plant your feet flat on the floor, and feel the connection between the soles of your feet and the ground. Close your eyes and imagine that your feet are growing roots and that these roots are reaching down, through the layers of flooring, all the way to the earth below and penetrating deeply into the soil. Imagine sending all your stress and anxiety down through these roots, releasing these negative sensations into the earth. Then imagine bringing up through the roots all the calming, soothing energy of the earth, in the same way as a tree soaks up water and nutrients. Allow the solid, quiet energy of the earth to come up through these roots and begin to fill your body from the legs up, until you're filled with calm earth energy. Then take a moment to sit quietly in the chair, just experiencing this sense of grounding.

Another grounding exercise is to sit on a straight-backed chair with your feet flat on the floor, and bring attention to your breath. As you inhale, begin to bring your breath right down into the bottom of your belly, but without forcing it. When you exhale, allow the belly to fall back naturally and the air to flow out without effort. Do this slowly, several times. Notice that as you breathe in, you feel like you're settling down into the chair. Notice that when you exhale, you're staying solid and grounded in the chair. As you breathe more deeply and slowly, you should begin to experience calmness and peace. You should feel more connected to the chair you're sitting in, and to the ground.

TRANSFERENCE OF ADDICTIONS

Ever since gastric bypass and lap-band surgery have become more common, a phenomenon known as the transference of addictions has been recognized. It's also called "cross addiction." People are saying it's a new occurrence but it's been around as long as there have been addictions because, essentially, all addictions are interchangeable.

Not that long ago, my office was situated upstairs from a 12 Step meeting place. On my way out at the end of the day, I'd see participants standing in front of the building during their break, puffing away on cigarettes and drinking extra-large coffees. It was clear to me then that they had transferred their alcohol addiction to cigarettes and coffee.

When overeating is no longer an option for the child within, it creates a gap that needs to be filled by something else. As an overeater, you have two choices: to turn to another addiction or become conscious of your emotional wound and see that it requires true healing. If you don't deal directly with the issues involved in your eating behavior, it's inevitable that you'll transfer your current addiction to some other one if, for example, surgery has made overeating impossible. The wound within compels the child to deal with it. The choice is whether to allow the child within to continue pursuing false solutions to her healing or to have the adult self take over this role and begin giving the child within what she really needs.

FOLLOWING YOUR DREAM: MEANING, PURPOSE, AND CONNECTION

My patient Eloise discovered a very interesting relationship between pursuing her dreams and binge eating. When she began to work on an art project that she'd always dreamed of doing but had never been able to pursue until she got into therapy, she noticed that the urge to binge dramatically decreased. The more she dealt with her wounds, the more she was able to work on her project and the less driven she was to binge eat. It wasn't a matter of self-control; she just lost the desire to overeat. By not being sidetracked by her binges, Eloise had more time for her project and, suddenly, she was thinner and living her artistic dream. A positive circle was created, where healing promoted pursuing her art, and this brought her freedom from the desire to binge, which further promoted living her dream.

While you're facing, grieving, and letting go of your wounds and beginning to find freedom from your eating, food, and weight problems, you'll start to find that time and space will open up so that you can explore your real wants and needs. When you've made the commitment to be responsible for your life and healing, you'll be less and less tempted to think that your happiness lies in the quick, easy, and false solution of addiction.

When, as an adult, you desire true fulfillment, you won't have to waste your energy on false solutions to the wounds of your childhood. Instead of busily feeding the bottomless pit of need created by your unaddressed wounds, or being led astray by the latest fad diet, you can begin to feed your soul. In my experience, it's love and connection with others, meaningful and productive work, enjoyable leisure, fulfilling creativity, and a sense of belonging to all living beings that will do this for you.

In any compulsive-addictive behavior pattern, the aims are always twofold: to be soothed or distracted from your unconscious pain, anger, or sadness from past losses and to find a substitute for the love and fulfillment that was lacking in your childhood. Addictive substances or behaviors can be stimulating and distracting, like gambling, shopping, overexercising, or overworking, or they can be soothing and anesthetizing, like alcohol or sedative drugs. Overeating is unique in that it can be soothing, distracting, or stimulating, depending on the type and amount of food eaten.

The problem with addiction is that all its effects are superficial and short lived, at which point your unresolved feelings and unmet needs begin to make themselves known again and the urges recur, in cravings for a snack, a drink, a shopping spree, or a trip to the casino.

When consciousness begins to grow within you, you'll be able to recognize and change your addictive behavior. As I said before, initially, you could have just finished a binge, for example, and then recognized that it wasn't what you really needed. As you become more conscious, you could next find yourself in the middle of a binge, suddenly aware of what you're doing. You can then say to yourself, "Wait a minute! This isn't what I really want." Recognizing that the addictive substance or activity has nothing to offer you, you'll be able to walk away from it without having to force yourself to do so. And by practicing ruthless compassion, the inner critic won't get a chance to sabotage the opportunity for learning by making the child within feel bad about you catching yourself mid-binge.

With consciousness, the decision to let go of the addictive behavior will be natural and easy. After you've "woken up" a few times in the middle of an eating, boozing, shopping, or gambling binge, your "consciousness muscle" will be strengthened and you'll become aware of what you're doing sooner and sooner in the process. With no self-criticism involved, you won't need to shut down the process. Eventually, as soon as you begin to feel the urge to binge, you'll be able to say to yourself, "No, I don't want this. It's bad a habit that's never made me feel better. In fact, it's always made me feel worse." With consciousness, you'll be able to see the urge for what it is—a misguided attempt at self-care—and you'll be able to stop it before the binge even starts.

As you work on healing your childhood wounds, nurturing the child within, pursuing your dreams, and developing conscious awareness, you'll move to the final stage of letting go of addiction: you'll stop having the urge to engage in the addiction almost entirely.

It might come back now and then, if you're triggered by a memory of a past hurt, overcome by some powerful emotions or if your consciousness slips momentarily. But, having healed the majority of your wounds and developed your consciousness, even these occasional urges will be easy to see for what they are: just reminders of an old, dysfunctional way of coping. From a combination of ruthless compassion and the conscious awareness that addiction isn't what you need, your adult self will be able to let go of the old pattern of compulsive behavior and obsessive thinking, and you'll be free to turn to what you really need.

In the healing and self-nurturing process, you'll discover what really brings happiness. The enduring fulfillment of engaging in meaningful relationships and activities creates a clear contrast to your compulsive eating. As Sigmund Freud said, we need "work, love and play" in our lives to be fulfilled as adults. I would add meaning, purpose, and connection and then I think you'd have everything you need for a good life.

When I was a youngster, I used to love to draw. I'd sit and sketch various things in my house: the potted plants, cups and saucers, my dog while she was sleeping. In pre-med, on my breaks from studying, I'd sketch the furniture and walls in my apartment. Drawing has always been something that I enjoyed, and eventually I saw that I'd gotten good at it without really trying. Time and repetition enabled me to develop a solid technique.

In fact, it took me years to learn to draw well, but my focus was on enjoying the experience. It's also taken me years to develop as a psychotherapist, and I continue to enjoy the process of learning this work. It bears repeating: everything worthwhile takes time. If you don't let the impatience of the child within pressure you for immediate gratification, you'll be rewarded by the deep fulfillment of something that's grown over time into a real skill, a meaningful relationship or a true understanding.

I've appreciated all the moments I've spent drawing, as they themselves were fulfilling. The *process* by which you develop your skills or your relationships is as important as the *goal* of the journey. In fact, there is no real end point. When will I be done learning as an artist or a therapist? When will a relationship be "just right?" There's no end, just a journey in which you deepen your enjoyment, commitment, and fulfillment with regard to whatever it is you're pursuing.

At some point, you might feel that you've gotten "good enough" at something or that you feel deeply contented in your relationship. Over time and with practice, you'll gain a sense of mastery and fulfillment from your work, love, and play, and a sense of meaning and connection in your life. There's never any need to aspire to perfection.

The internalized parent pushes the child within to be perfect, but nothing will ever satisfy this part of the psyche that is incapable of being pleased. When the child feels pressure to meet impossible parental expectations, she'll give up in despair or act out in defiance, and you'll be unhappy. With the adult in charge, you'll see that being "good enough" at things is all you need for success. Sure, sometimes you'll want to excel because it feels good to strive for greatness and to get there, but you also need to know that you can have a good life even when you're not "the best."

Human beings aren't capable of perfection, and pursuing this false goal only leads to frustration and a sense of inadequacy or failure. The warrior within must combat the lie of perfectionism, and the child within must heed the adult who knows to be content with doing the best she can, whether she's up at the top or somewhere in the middle. In this way, fulfillment is possible.

The pursuit of perfection also promotes addiction. For example, if you're trying to get to "the perfect weight," rather than a healthy weight that's right for your age, lifestyle, and body type, you're doomed to fail. Pushing yourself to reach an unreasonable goal will cause the child within to sabotage your efforts at dieting. It's likely that you'll start to eat more than you did before, to compensate for the deprivation and to comfort yourself from the shame or disappointment over your "failure."

When you strive to please the internalized parent you're doomed to fail. Even when you're at the top, this voice will tell you that it's still not good enough. If you achieve your goal of the "perfect weight" and the negative self-talk is saying that you're "flabby" and should be more toned, that you need to do something about your cellulite or that you won't be able to keep the weight off, in no time at all you'll be gaining the weight back.

I have a very bright young patient, Clarisse, a graduate student in history, whom I've been seeing in therapy for a few years. She's extremely gifted, but is dominated by a perfectionist internalized parent that tells her that she's only acceptable if she's the best in her class. When she first started therapy, if she'd get 98 percent on a test and someone else got 99 percent, the internalized parent would criticize her for having failed. Clarisse constantly struggled in her ability to function; not just at school but in every aspect of her life. Through therapy, she came to recognize and reject the false demands of perfection and be content with the high level of success she was able to achieve.

The true dreams in your life come out of adult wants, and not from a parental "should." It's easy to know what you want, once you take the time to get in touch with your true adult needs and feelings and open your mind to what's possible for you. The child within may be afraid to dream because of fear of failure or because she feels that she's "not good enough," but she's just responding to inner messages telling her that she's inadequate or undeserving or that the world won't support her dreams. A realistic adult attitude will help you see that these parental messages are untrue and that success in life is neither guaranteed nor impossible but dependent on hard work, the passage of time, and a bit of luck.

In imagining what's possible for you, a balance of realism and positivity is the ideal approach. You mustn't be so unrealistic that you strive for things that are clearly out of your reach, but equally, you shouldn't be so negative that you rule out too many possibilities. Ruthless compassion will enable you to see yourself and your options with clarity and without self-criticism, and will help you recognize your assets and your challenges. Being in reality while pursuing your dreams will make them much more likely to come true, whereas being stuck in overly optimistic (child fantasy) or overly pessimistic (parental negativity or child despair) beliefs or expectations will stymie your chances of success.

Being in the process of pursuing real dreams of meaningful relationships, fulfilling work, and enjoyable pastimes will enable you to gain a sense of fulfillment. This fulfillment will counteract the compulsion to use food and weight in order to meet the needs of the child within. One you feel fulfilled, you'll have no need or desire to overfill yourself with false solutions. Real fulfillment will come from following your dreams.

People who overeat do so because they're bored, lonely, angry, needy, or frustrated. They eat because they have wounds that are calling out to be healed or because there's something missing in their lives. If you were once slim and fit and are now overweight, perhaps you've misplaced your dream. Perhaps you've lost sight of what's most important to your happiness and well-being. You may have a loving family, a good job and friends, but you've forgotten what you really want. Maybe in the hustle and bustle of your life you've just let it go.

Perhaps you've rationalized that your life is fine the way it is. You've been settling for a so-so life because, by comparison, it's a far cry better than the childhood you lived through. If you're more than a little bit overweight, though, it means that you've compromised too much. Getting back in touch with what you really want and pursuing your dream even if it seems, to the critical parental voice, foolish or trivial, is what will make the difference between a truly happy and fulfilled life, and a so-so life in which you overeat to compensate for what's missing.

Becoming Your Optimal Self

There's a best version of each of us that I call the "optimal self." This is the self who has grown into a fully functioning adult. She's able to call forward a powerful inner warrior; she's gotten the child within to take its proper place in the background of her psyche, she's in touch with her inner wisdom, and she's banished the internalized parent to the graveyard for old, unheeded opponents. Once you've done your healing work and are fully engaged in loving and caring for the child within, you can aspire to this way of being.

The optimal self is you at your very best. You aren't in competition with anyone else and you don't need to be compared to anyone else. This is the way of being that's best for you and the version of you that can contribute the most to the world.

The optimal self is free of addiction and empowered to pursue her true dreams. She's fully responsible for her choices and honest with herself, with an attitude of ruthless compassion. She doesn't settle for a "bad deal" with a friend, a partner, or at work because she knows that this will erode her confidence and could lead to anxiety, depression, or addiction. She doesn't settle for "the next best" of anything, but holds out for what she knows is right. She doesn't make choices out of fear but out of conscious awareness of what she really wants.

She trusts herself, and knows that she can pursue her goals and take care of herself, no matter what comes along. She sees people as companions on her journey, but not as "the answer" to her problems. She's neither overly needy nor exploitative; she feels free to give and receive love and friendship and appreciates the contribution people make to her life.

She listens to her inner wisdom and trusts her intuition. She knows the difference between the voice of the wise one within and the devious inner critic who masquerades as the voice of reason.

The optimal self is awake and aware; she knows and accepts herself. Because she takes good care of herself, she doesn't waste her time being angry or frustrated. When others behave badly toward her, she effectively deals with these people with integrity, clarity, and strength. She understands that the practice of ruthless compassion enables her to exercise realistic options in her dealings with others.

Your optimal self has more to offer than the wounded version of yourself because your self-love will overflow to others and they'll benefit from your loving kindness. With clear boundaries, an autonomous attitude, and self-confident entitlement, your optimal self will model to others a better way to live.

The optimal self is neither isolated nor withdrawn, but she's content being alone. She's comfortable in her own skin and doesn't need anyone else to entertain her or distract her from her feelings. She's never desperate for company or attention, and she'll never compromise herself or "sell out" in order to keep someone around.

It's never preferable for her to be in a relationship just for the sake of having someone; she'll only choose to be with a friend or partner if he or she adds value to her life. She enjoys her own company, taking time to attend to the needs that only she can fulfill. The optimal self loves and enjoys other people, but she recognizes that they're not responsible for the nurturing or healing of the child within. She learns from her friends and loved ones, shares with them and collaborates with them toward mutual goals.

The optimal self knows that those who love her will do so regardless of whether or not she fulfills all their expectations, and that those whose threaten to punish or abandon her if she can't or won't please them have no real love to give. She understands that people who set such terms only see her as an object for the purposes of their own gratification. She knows that she has the right to say "no" when she wants to, and that those who love her will continue to love her, even when she doesn't agree to all of their wishes.

The optimal self is an excellent parent because she has clear expectations, gives unconditional love, sets straightforward limits, and gives appropriate consequences. In relationships, she's honest and open about her needs and feelings and she doesn't fear her partner's responses to her requests. She understands that how someone responds to the expression of her needs and feelings gives her important information about whether they care. She's clear about what she can't accept in a relationship and what she can't live without. Because she doesn't settle for having less than what she needs and she doesn't tolerate unacceptable behavior, she never carries around the hurt, anger, or resentment that could lead to frustration, passive-aggression, or addiction.

The optimal self knows that those who love you do so because of *who you are* and are genuinely interested in you and glad for your success. They'll never try to hold you back or keep you down for their own purposes. She knows that there are those who only pretend to love you and that these individuals benefit from *what you do for them.* They're jealous or resentful about what you have and what you've accomplished.

The optimal self knows how to deal with hurtful behavior on the part of others. She understands that when she's done something to upset friends, they can present their needs and feelings to her in a reasonable and respectful manner. If someone insults her, engages in psychological game playing or is passive-aggressive, she knows that it's not about her. She recognizes that people who behave badly do so from their own wounds and not because of something she's done. She also knows that she's human and vulnerable and that cruelty can cause her pain, even when she's clear that it has nothing to do with her.

She also knows that it's not enough to say to herself, "this isn't about me." She realizes that she must defend herself from attacks and protect herself from further attacks. She sees the truth about the people who are badly behaved toward her and considers her options, deciding on the best choice for each situation. While someone is behaving in a hurtful manner, she can decide to extricate herself from the situation, she can stand up for herself and confront them about the unacceptability of their behavior, or she can provide consequences for the behavior after the fact. Another option is no longer choosing to have this person in her life.

The optimal self realizes that having an explanation for someone's bad behavior doesn't make it acceptable. She knows that adults are accountable for their actions and always have a choice about how they behave. She sees that understanding why someone behaves badly doesn't make the behavior less hurtful. She knows that she can choose only to associate with people who take responsibility for themselves; those who are kind to begin with or those who'll face up to their bad behavior and decide to change for the better.

The optimal self isn't afraid of failure because she doesn't see it as inevitable or permanent. She's able to learn from her mistakes without self-criticism and sees her failures as opportunities for growth. She's equally unafraid of success, trusting that she can handle all that success brings to her life. She sees her assets and her deficits clearly without false modesty or false pride. She's always learning about what she's capable of, what she needs to work on in her personal growth and which false dreams to let go of. She's objective about the people in her life and doesn't choose her friends or partner based on the potential she sees in them but on the way they behave, right now. She's fully grounded in reality and isn't carrying any illusions about what she herself, or anyone else is able to achieve.

In the workplace, the optimal self values her contribution and expects to be reasonably rewarded for it. She understands that not receiving credit for her work or allowing her ideas to be stolen is damaging to her as a person. She understands that commitment, loyalty, integrity, and creative collaboration are what make a positive work environment and that a toxic workplace should be avoided, no matter how lucrative it might be. She knows that no amount of money can compensate for being disrespected, undervalued, exploited, or abused by a supervisor or colleague.

The optimal self loves her body, whatever shape it's in, and appreciates what her body can do for her. She accepts her physical limitations but doesn't settle for a minimum level of health. She exercises to stay fit and to remind herself that she's a physical being who can't just live in her head. The rejection of the body is not for the optimal self. She respects her body by nourishing it with wholesome foods. She avoids toxic chemicals, drugs, and food additives because she's conscious that what she ingests has a significant impact on her physical and emotional well-being.

The optimal self lives at the optimal weight for her body type, age, culture, and environment. She enjoys her food without being obsessive about it, and without any compulsive eating behaviors. She isn't concerned about being "too fat" or trying to be unrealistically thin. She's free from addiction to food or anything else because she's put her wounds behind her and has moved beyond the pursuit of false solutions to her healing and nurturing.

The optimal self is healthy in body, mind, emotions, sexuality, and spirit; she's in balance within herself and in her world. She adds benefit to her environment because she's overflowing with positive energy. The better care she takes of herself, the more she has to offer to others. She understands that self-care isn't selfishness and that self-esteem isn't arrogance.

She knows that it's good to be proud of herself and her accomplishments and that anyone who has a problem with this is jealous of her deserved success. She knows that those who criticize her for doing well are angry and unhappy, and that she should never have to diminish herself in order to be less threatening to someone else.

The optimal self isn't "nice," but she's kind. She isn't a pleaser, but she's caring and compassionate. She's not preoccupied with what others think or say about her. If people are critical, she knows it's because of their own unhappiness and wounds. On the other hand, she's responsive to constructive feedback and is open to changing something about herself if it makes sense. She isn't rigid or defensive, because self-acceptance includes always wanting to grow.

She's self-motivated and passionate about her goals. She's not dependent on others' approval or afraid of their critiques. She always strives to do her best but has nothing to prove. She's comfortable with who she is and has a relaxed, confident, and pleasant attitude.

The optimal self enjoys collaborating on projects with others. She soaks up learning without shame over any ignorance or errors. She has realistic expectations of herself and others. She respects others and expects respect from them. The optimal self owns her power, but it's the power to live her best life and to pursue her goals rather than power over anyone or anything.

The optimal self is calm and peaceful but never bored. She easily balances being productive and taking time to relax and recharge. She's able to enjoy her moments of happiness and to confidently cope with life's difficulties.

If you read all of the above and thought, "I can't get there. That's not possible for me," it's either the lie of the inner critic or the fear of the child within. Don't give up so easily. If you doubt that you can become your optimal self, it could be because you're attached to your old identity and afraid of change.

Developing a conscious, empowered adult identity, banishing the inner critic, healing and nurturing the child within, and practicing ruthless compassion will naturally bring forward your optimal self. Here's a visualization to help you get in touch with your optimal self.

VISUALIZATION 4: THE COCOON—BECOMING YOUR OPTIMAL SELF

In this visualization, you'll be taking symbolic steps toward becoming your optimal self. In your comfortable, straight-backed chair, plant your feet, close your eyes, connect with the rhythms of your breathing, and relax.

Imagine yourself standing in a large, quiet and beautiful summer garden. Feel your bare feet connected to the earth. Feel the gentle, cooling breezes against your skin and look around at the ring of tall trees surrounding the space, making it safe and private.

You're standing in the center of this garden, surrounded by flowers that are gently swaying in the breeze. The strong sun is relaxing your muscles and warming you deeply. You begin to perspire, but instead of droplets running down your face and body, magical, wispy tendrils of a gossamer-like substance are emerging from your pores.

The breeze picks up and begins to swirl around you, and the fine tendrils coming off your body are being wrapped around you. The swirling breezes are wrapping you in layer upon layer of these fine strands. Soon, you're completely covered in a soft, loose, almost opaque cocoon. All you can see is the light of the garden.

From within this cocoon, a transformation is going to take place. You're about to become your optimal self. Connect with your feelings and let go of all judgments about yourself. You're completely safe and secure. Surrender to this positive experience of change.

First, within the cocoon, feel your physical self transformed into the most fit and healthy version of your body possible. You are strong and flexible, energized yet calm. Your body feels awake and alive. As you experience and enjoy this new physical self, a layer of the cocoon falls off and is blown away by the breeze.

Next, feel your emotions flowing freely. You're peaceful and confident, no longer attached to any feelings from the past. You're free to experience all the emotions of the present, including joy, wonder, and love. Your heart is fully open and can be filled again and again, only to overflow with loving kindness. You aren't afraid of your feelings because you know that you're more powerful than any one of them. As you stand here with a full and easy heart, another layer of the cocoon floats away.

Now, feel your creative self becoming inspired and uplifted. You're free to pursue your dreams and to make your voice heard. You're able to make your mark on the world and to create the best life for yourself and others. As you stand here, reveling in your creative power, another layer of the cocoon floats away.

Next, experience your mental and intellectual self blossoming. You feel mentally enriched and fulfilled. Your intellect is engaged and utilized. You experience clarity and a depth of understanding, wisdom, and knowledge. You're conscious and aware. As you stand there in all your mental acuity, another layer of the cocoon comes off and is carried away by the breeze.

Feel, now, the capacity within yourself to connect with others in a meaningful way. Feel the ability to form loving, constructive relationships and build a sense of community. Feel a deeper sense of belonging as well as a feeling of autonomy and self-reliance. Experience a sense of clear boundaries and the knowledge that you'll give and receive nothing but respect. As you stand there, feeling a strong sense of belonging, one more layer of the cocoon falls away.

Now, feel a sense of oneness with all living things. You're connected to everyone and everything. You feel a sense of wholeness and safety, knowing that you're one with the universe. You're comforted by the awareness that you're an integral part of all life. Standing there, feeling this deep sense of connectedness to everything, a layer of the cocoon floats away.

Experience, now, your sexual being fully alive and in balance, with the joy and delight of your body and sensuality rediscovered. Feel a sense of safety, power, and choice, as well as playfulness and curiosity. Notice how all shame, guilt, and fear have gone away, and that your sexuality is innocent and mature, open, but with good boundaries, gentle, and empowered. As you stand there in all your sexual power and glory, another layer of the cocoon comes off.

Now, standing in the garden with only the thinnest membrane between you and the outside world, take a moment to savor this experience of transformation. Imagine that each of the transformed aspects of yourself have created tiny seeds of life energy. Imagine that these seeds are planted in your belly, and that they're beginning to sprout. They grow into shoots, and then develop into supple stalks that intertwine with one another until a great braided plant made of positive energy is lined up along your spine, with branches going up into your arms and head and roots going all the way down your legs.

This tree of transformation lives deep within you. Each part of the trunk must be strong for the tree to be in balance. Feel this energy tree within you, strong and tall, where all the aspects of yourself—the physical, emotional, creative, mental, relational, spiritual, and sexual—are in harmony with each other.

As you stand in the meadow with this tree of transformation growing within you, the last layer of the cocoon floats away. You contain at this very moment the potential within you to be the very best version of yourself that you can be. Take a moment to savor this experience and when you're ready, return to the here and now.

7

Reclaiming Your Power, Sensuality, and Sexuality

Sexuality, Inner Wounds, and Healing

My patient Billie was the recipient of inappropriate sexual attention when she was too young to know how to deal with it. She was molested at age seven by a friend of the family over a period of several months. On top of this, when she began to develop sexually at age 13, she was made to feel uncomfortable about her changing body. Her father and an uncle by marriage used to look at her in ways that made her feel ashamed. These experiences violated her boundaries and she ended up with significant wounds with regard to her body and her sexuality.

Sadly, Billie is one of many women in my practice who've experienced some type of sexual trauma. These women were ogled, fondled, or abused by relatives, neighbors, teachers, group leaders, clerics, or coaches. Some were very little when it happened, while others were preteens or teens. I've also worked with men who were sexually abused as children. All of these individuals felt powerless to resist or stop the abuse.

As children, they were too young to understand what was happening, and even as teens, they weren't capable of making responsible, informed decisions about their sexuality. Some of these individuals passively went along with the abuse because they were so starved for love and desperate for any sort of positive attention that even this bad type of attention seemed better than nothing. This decision is typical of child logic. It makes sense at the time but has unfortunate consequences (including guilt and shame) later on.

Almost all of the women in my practice who were sexually traumatized as children have an eating disorder, as do some of the men. Many of them are overeaters (although a few have suffered from anorexia or bulimia) and all of them have enormous shame and anxiety around their sexuality. Whether as helpless victims or naïvely colluding with the perpetrator, they grew up feeling bad about themselves. Most of them believe today that they were in some way responsible for what happened, that they should have been able to stop it, and that they were bad because they didn't.

Some of them were told by the perpetrator to keep the abuse a secret; some were threatened with violence if they spoke up. Keeping this secret made them feel complicit with the abuse, which brought on more shame. Some of them knew that there was no point in telling their parents, and some sought parental help even when evidence from past experience showed them that they wouldn't be believed or protected. Their parents' unwillingness to believe them or defend them was seen as a reflection of their own worthlessness. Most of them developed the unconscious belief that it would be futile to try to escape from any future abuse.

Some of the women who'd been able to tell their mothers what had happened to them were accused of "seducing" their abusers; others were met with denial or indifference. As a result, these women felt abandoned, powerless, and undeserving of protection. Many of the women grew up feeling that physically, they must have been too tempting for their abusers, and that they needed to change their bodies so as to be less seductive and therefore safe from future abuse.

Many of the women who experienced sexual abuse during childhood or adolescence have been unconsciously using their extra weight as a means of avoiding their sexuality. While many overweight women have no history of sexual abuse, a majority of women who have a history of childhood sexual abuse will eventually develop some type of eating disorder, and many of them will be overweight.

Sexuality is a necessary and wonderful part of a woman's life, but because it was forced on these women when they were too young to understand it or to defend themselves, and because no one protected or defended them, their sexuality was wounded. If they want to be whole as women, they must heal their sexual wounds and reclaim their sexuality as the positive and natural thing it ought to be.

Billie is similar to many women with a history of sexual trauma. She's been unconsciously exempting herself from the arena of adult sexuality. Being overweight, she's tried to neutralize her body by eliminating its contours, and she's avoided sexual relationships for years. Whether gay or straight, young or old, women with a history of sexual abuse or inappropriate sexual attention often feel intolerably vulnerable in their bodies. The women who become heavy can disconnect from their physical selves and avoid having to deal with sex.

The feelings of shame that Billie experienced as a result of the boundary violations she experienced while young have now been transferred to her weight. Like other women with a similar history, she sees the extra weight as embarrassing, and this causes her to feel even more disconnected from her body.

Billie, and all the other women who've experienced similar trauma, must see that the extra weight is a response to their wounds as opposed to a mark of shame. Letting go of feelings of shame and powerlessness around their bodies will be a necessary part of healing their sexuality.

Shame is such a negative experience that it requires great effort to eliminate it from the psyche. In dealing with any type of sexual boundary violation the support, guidance, and expertise of a trained psychotherapist can help you navigate the difficult path of healing. The first thing you'll discover is that it wasn't your fault, your body is not seductive, and you didn't deserve the abuse.

A skilled and experienced therapist can help you to inhabit your adult self. You'll be able to spend time connecting with the child within, letting her know that the trauma she experienced was a reflection of the perpetrator, not her. The adult can tell the child within that if she wasn't protected from this abuse, it was due to the limited capacity of her parents or guardians and not because she lacked value or deserved it. Your therapist can help you see that even if you went along with the abuse, it wasn't your fault because at the time you were incapable of making conscious decisions with regard to your sexuality, and perhaps because your desperate need for love was being exploited by the abuser.

A therapist can help you see that in every case of sexual activity between an adult and a child, the adult is the one with the power and the one who is taking advantage of the child. You'll learn that your body was never to blame for what happened to you. The abuse was a result of disturbed individuals being unable to control their inappropriate urges and impulses.

Through therapy, Billie has been able to grieve the loss of her sexual innocence. She's learning to accept herself and her body and is beginning to see sexuality as something over which she can have power and choice. She knows that today, she's free to say "no." She understands that sexuality isn't about being subject to another person's desires and demands, but about mutual respect and caring, where her feelings and needs matter.

She's seeing that sex doesn't have to be equated with exploitation but also that it doesn't automatically mean love. Therapy is showing her that when someone is attracted to her, she's done nothing wrong and isn't responsible for having seduced them. She's learning that every adult is responsible for their sexuality, and that her choices are a reflection of her desires rather than her worth.

Through therapy, Billie is seeing that she's valuable and worth protecting. This newfound self-worth will enable her to protect and defend herself in the future in a way that her loved ones wouldn't or couldn't in the past. She's reclaiming her healthy sexuality and rather than feeling like a helpless victim. Billie is becoming someone who has freedom of choice. Ultimately, she'll begin to let go of the extra weight that she no longer needs.

While you're in the process of healing the wounds of your childhood and letting go of compulsive eating, you can reenter the sexual arena any time you want, whatever you weigh. You can be attractive and desirable at any weight. If you let go of shame around your body and sexuality, you'll radiate confidence and prospective partners will show interest in you.

There's no physical reason why an overweight woman can't have good sex. If someone desires you and is interested in engaging in a sexual relationship with you, it's only the inner critic who says that your weight should prohibit this. If the child within trusts that you know what you're doing and that you'll keep her safe, there's no reason for you to use your weight as an excuse to avoid intimacy.

It's up to you how you choose to express your sexuality, so you should spend some time getting in touch with what you want and what you feel comfortable with. Most importantly, you should keep checking in with yourself, stay true to yourself and never go along with anything that feels wrong even if someone is pushing you to do it. Your sexuality is yours, and although sometimes you might use it to give pleasure to someone, you should never be a pleaser.

If you abandon yourself sexually, you risk retriggering the old trauma. Those of you who've struggled with sexual abuse or boundary violations in the past need to feel empowered around your present-day sexuality. Make sure that what you do, when you do it, how you do it, and with whom you do it is up to you. Working with a therapist on facing and grieving the loss of innocence and the traumas you experienced, letting go of the guilt, shame, and anger deep within you and reclaiming your healthy sexuality are all part of becoming your optimal self.

Sensuality and Weight

As a little girl, Emily, a 57-year-old nurse, sometimes complained to her mother about feeling sad, and her mother would always respond that she didn't think Emily was feeling sad at all. This was confusing to Emily because at the time, she really did feel sad. Still, she trusted her mother and wanted her approval, so she believed what her mother said.

The truth was that her mother didn't want to hear about Emily being sad because it would have meant that she'd have to make the effort to help her daughter. Emily's mother didn't want to do this so she told her daughter, "you're not sad, honey, you're just tired." As a result, Emily grew up unclear about the difference between "sad" and "tired."

This wasn't the only feeling Emily's mother refused to acknowledge. When Emily said that she was angry, her mother told her that hunger was making her cranky, and offered her a snack. As she grew up, Emily became more comfortable intellectualizing her experiences rather than trying to sort out her confusing emotions. Having her feelings negated during childhood caused Emily to grow into an emotionally disconnected adult.

You live in your body, so you need to feel connected to it. Many people live in their heads, especially intelligent women who've been made to feel bad about their bodies or confused about their feelings. They're out of touch with their bodily sensations, their physical needs, and their feelings, and they're prone to overanalyzing their experiences.

It's also likely that you'd be disconnected from your physical self if you've been shamed while growing up, either from having experienced physical boundary violations, or by having been constantly subject to the contempt of your caretakers. The experience of trauma at a young age frequently leads to what's called "dissociation" or feelings of detachment from yourself or your environment.

For example, when a child is being molested, it's an unbearable experience. She has nowhere to go and is unable to defend herself. She feels shock, fear, pain, and rage at this violation, but has no choice except to submit. The abuse is intolerable so she "goes away," disconnecting from reality and imagining herself in another place, where this awful thing isn't happening to her.

There are mild forms of dissociation, like daydreaming when you're bored, and more serious forms of dissociation, such as "tuning out" or "going blank." The most severe type is dissociative identity disorder, or what's commonly known as "multiple personality."

If you're someone who grew up with confusing messages about your emotions, ongoing parental contempt, or assaults to your physical boundaries, you'll probably be overly aware of what you're thinking and under-aware of your sensations and emotions. You might even sometimes "go away." When you're out of touch with your body and emotions, it's easier to live in your mind where you feel safe.

A woman who has grown up with physical, sexual, or emotional abuse could have symptoms of post-traumatic stress disorder, or PTSD; one symptom of which is dissociation when under stress. In the absence of a conscious adult identity, the child within defends herself from intolerable emotions by intellectualizing or emotionally shutting down.

A woman who was sexually abused as a child may have trouble tolerating certain bodily sensations because they might remind her of what she experienced during the abuse. She won't want to rub lotion onto her body because it might remind her of an inappropriate caress; she won't want to take long showers because being naked for more than a few minutes could bring back a sense of vulnerability and cause her to feel anxious; she might become very overweight in order to transform her body into something asexual and non-threatening.

Not every sufferer of PTSD overeats but those who do, do so in order to numb their feelings and take away their pain, fear, and anger. Sadly, while the overeating helps a sufferer of PTSD push away threatening emotions, it also serves to keep her disconnected from what she needs in order to heal.

During a binge, you can be so caught up in the child-driven compulsion to self-soothe and bury your pain that you'll be disconnected from your physical sensations. You might not remember how much or even what you ate during an episode of binge eating. You'll barely taste what you're eating and you won't register that you're becoming full. Eventually, you'll get to the point of feeling overfull, a sensation unpleasant enough to make you choose to maintain your disconnection from your physical sensations.

When you don't feel connected to your body, you might not even be aware of your actual size. You could have a distorted idea of your body, believing that you're smaller or bigger than you really are. You might want to avoid acknowledging your size and shape out of fear of the criticisms of the internalized parent, or fear of feeling vulnerable.

This disconnect from the physical is a psychological defense mechanism whose aim is to protect you from memories of trauma, or from feelings of pain, fear, self-reproach, or shame. Unfortunately this defense mechanism only leads to self-alienation and doesn't fend off the self-judgment. It certainly does nothing to address the trauma.

If you're emotionally confused or shut down, you'll need to make time to reconnect with your feelings so that you can be a whole person, living in your body and not just in your head. If you have a history of emotional, physical, or sexual abuse, it is essential that you face, grieve, and let go of your wounds so that you no longer fear or avoid your feelings.

Because sexual abuse is such a profound insult to the child's being, the grieving process may be more intense and lengthy than that which you'd do for any other childhood wounds, but it can be completed. By grieving fully, ideally with therapeutic support, you'll be able to understand that connecting to your emotions and experiencing your bodily sensations is not only safe but will provide you with a richer, more satisfying existence. You'll finally be able to return to the body you separated from during the abuse. The body that once was a dangerous place, harboring painful memories and frightening sensations will finally be your home.

Our society also is to blame for how you feel about your body. It promotes unreasonable expectations of thinness to which the child within reacts with rebellion or despair. I believe that the increase in obesity is partly due to the increasing pressure young girls and women experience as a result of the media messages they're constantly absorbing.

"Be thinner. Be much thinner," you're told, first by the outer parents (the media) and then by the internalized one. For some of you, the child within will first try to please this demanding voice. She'll eat very little, sometimes even becoming anorexic, in order to live up to this impossible expectation of perfection. For some women, the child within is convinced that she could never be thin enough so she doesn't even try; in other women, the child sabotages the attempt out of spite. Many women are split in two, binge eating to feed the needy child within and then purging in order to please the inner critic, in the disordered eating of bulimia.

Reacting to societal pressure to change your body only makes you disconnect from it that much more. Instead of enjoying your body, it becomes a "project" to perfect, a symbol of your failure or an entity you're at war with. Rather than appreciating the good fortune of physical health and mobility, you agonize about your imperfect body as though it were an inanimate object attached to your head.

A patient of mine told me a horrifying story several years ago. It was about a Toronto elementary school where the girls were going on diets at age seven or eight because the "popular" boys, who were in Grades 6 and 7, demanded that the girls they dated weigh no more than 100 pounds.

Twelve-year-old boys were putting weight restrictions on their potential girlfriends, but more mind boggling was how readily the girls were willing to comply. They were limiting their food intake in Grades 2 or 3 in preparation for dates that wouldn't take place for several years. I'm appalled by this story. Societal pressure was making these girls believe that dieting in order to be acceptable to boys was an appropriate thing to do.

Adult women aren't faring much better. Many of you constantly compare your body to other women. You feel good about yourself if you're thinner, so you try to eat less in order to win the unspoken competition. Some of you overeat, feeling you can't win. You think, "why bother?"

Being extremely thin has become a competitive sport among women of all ages and types, often inducing anorexia, bulimia, or obesity. Men also judge women by their weight and many will reject a woman simply because of her weight. They might not be turned off by a larger woman but because of the possible social repercussions, they avoid being with someone heavy.

It's crucial that you accept your body as it is, right now, no matter what its size and shape. The media and popular culture want to appropriate your body but you're free to take it back. Comparing yourself with others is a self-destructive pursuit because there will always be someone smaller (and someone larger) than you. Everyone is different and you don't know why someone might be thin. They might have a fast metabolism. Maybe they're anorexic, or ill.

People fall into one of three basic body types, described in the 1940s by an American psychologist Dr. William Sheldon: endomorph, mesomorph, or ectomorph, otherwise known as heavy build, medium build, and slim build. No matter how much or how little you eat, you're born with a predisposition to a particular body type, and trying to diet yourself down from a mesomorph to an ectomorph, for example, will put your body and psyche under tremendous stress. There are also changes in a woman's body through her life cycle, with menopause being a stage where her body begins to carry weight differently than before. When a 50-year-old woman tries to compete with the 20-year-olds for who can be most thin, she's fighting a battle that even if she wins, she loses, because of the stress she puts on her mind and body.

There's a lot of societal support for being thin but very little for enjoying your physical self. Sadly, even in the 21st century, sensuality is seen as something questionable. We live in a time of absurd extremes, where an excess of meaningless sexual acting out coexists with old-fashioned prudishness. Whereas casual, even hard-core sexuality is now so common as to be unremarkable, sensuality is often looked at as self-indulgent, sinful, or even perverted. In reality, sensuality is simply the natural enjoyment of your body and physical sensations.

Whether it's taking a bubble bath, getting a massage, sharing a warm hug, stroking the soft fur of a pet, or holding hands with someone, sensuality is good for your body and soul. Touch triggers the release of endorphins, the neurotransmitter chemicals in the brain that cause feelings of pleasure, well-being, and relaxation.

Sensuality decreases anxiety and reduces stress. Even a brief hug causes the release of the bonding hormone oxytocin (which is also released during breastfeeding, facilitating the maternal-child connection), resulting in a positive emotional experience. There's also a connection between the release of oxytocin and the body's ability to lose weight more easily. Intuitively it makes sense; when you feel good in your body, it's easier to become healthier. You can see how intimately emotions and physical sensations are linked.

On the other hand, cortisol, a hormone that's released under stress, makes it more difficult for you to lose weight. The release of cortisol actually causes fat to be deposited in the tissues. It's an adaptation from the time of "fight or flight," when humans needed reserves of fat to flee a predator or defend themselves against an enemy. High stress keeps cortisol levels high; however, decreasing stress through the enjoyment of your sensuality will release pleasurable, relaxing endorphins and oxytocin and will decrease cortisol levels, all of which will enable you to lose weight more easily. It's good for your health to be sensual, and sensuality can be enjoyed in many ways that aren't sexual. It's up to you how you choose to bring more sensuality into your life.

As a conscious, responsible adult, you're entitled to feel comfortable in your body. You don't have to be afraid of wearing a clingy outfit, dancing with abandon, receiving a massage, or sunbathing on a beach. You'll understand that being sensual isn't the same as looking for sex. You can be clear about this distinction and confident that you can protect and defend yourself from inappropriate attention.

As an overweight woman, you might have been made to feel like you don't have the right to be sensual. According to some, only thin women "deserve" to enjoy their bodies, as though a woman is only allowed to take pleasure in her body if someone else gets to enjoy looking at it or touching it as well. That's absurd. No one should be deprived of the enjoyment, comfort, and touch she needs, whether it's a luxurious facial, a sensuous soak in a tub, or a loving embrace.

You're entitled to enjoy your body, whatever size or shape you are. Positive experiences of sensuality can help to heal any shame you're carrying. The innocent and respectful enjoyment of your physicality can transform your body from the repository of trauma and shame into the precious vehicle in which you live, move, and love.

Being more in touch with your physical self will enable you to recognize that you're similar to all the other living beings on the planet, and as a result of being more grounded in your physical self, you'll feel more connected to all life and more responsible for how you interact with the physical world.

It's hard to overeat when you're in touch with your body. Healing your wounds from the past will help heal your sensuality and healing your sensuality will help heal your disordered eating. When you're in touch with your body, you'll know when you feel full. You'll learn what foods make your body feel good, strong, and light and which ones make you feel heavy, achy, and dull.

Being in your body could also possibly help with your intuitive abilities. We all have a "gut sense" that may very well be connected to the physical network of nerves, or "plexus," located in the abdomen. When you're in touch with your body, you'll be more in touch with what your "gut sense" is trying to tell you, and this information will be very helpful.

If you trust your intuition, what I also call the "wise one within," your body will no longer be the battleground where the war of fat versus thin is waged. If you reclaim your sensuality, your body can be enjoyed and celebrated. If you're able to reconnect with your sensuality, you'll be more connected to your joy and your power, and therefore that much closer to letting go of compulsive eating and the need to be overweight.

CREATIVITY AND EMPOWERMENT

In one of the creativity and empowerment workshops that I run, a woman named Florence always used to say, "I'm not really good at art," as she was about to share a drawing with the group. Florence was a pianist and hadn't done much visual art. More to the point, her internalized parent had been telling her that unless she's instantly good at something, she'll never be able to do it well and therefore shouldn't bother trying.

She was terrified to take creative risks because her inner critic might disapprove of what she'd attempted. In reality, the women who participate in the workshop have told me that doing different types of creative exercises has helped them with their own particular form of creativity. The filmmaker in the group developed a fresh perspective, the interior designer was inspired to create some new designs, and the blocked writer was able to resume work on her novel.

Being creative in other ways supports your main form of creativity, proving that you don't have to buy into the false messages of the inner critic. Not being familiar with a medium doesn't mean you'll be bad at it. It just means you'll be inexperienced, which can often bring a lovely freshness and spontaneity to your work. It's important to know that for your own enjoyment and enrichment, you can be creative in whatever way you like, and no critic, whether internal or external, should prevent you from doing so.

In the same workshop, a woman named Elaina had difficulty staying with a creative project and completing it; she suffered from a lack of follow-through. For her, things had always come easily, and she'd never had to apply herself. She was a sculptor until a back injury forced her to give this up, and she came to the workshop feeling lost. She'd always done her art from the perspective of a playful, spontaneous child and had never learned adult discipline or sacrifice. Once she was injured and things no longer came easily, she got stuck. She'd turned to compulsive eating as a way to soothe her frustration.

Elaina learned that being creative isn't just about playing, but is a balance of the child's spontaneity and the adult's disciplined self-application. The child within might provide the spark of inspiration for a creative project but it's the adult self who carries it to completion, all the while making sure that the inner critic isn't sabotaging the process. As Elaina began to develop her adult identity, she slowly started getting better at following through with the creative projects given as homework for the workshop each week. When her creativity was flowing freely, she had less and less desire to overeat.

The critical parent in Florence's psyche was telling her that she was going to fail, and this made the child within feel hopeless and helpless. She feared humiliation, expecting the people in her life to echo the critic in her head. Anticipating a negative response from those who viewed her creative projects, she'd always make a disclaimer before showing her work to the group. In Elaina's case, the child within always brought creative inspiration to a project, but there was never enough adult energy to follow it through to completion. When it was time to share the homework, she'd present incomplete drawings and unedited writing assignments.

A child is a natural initiator, but isn't good at finishing things. She's impulsive and spontaneous, willing to be innovative and take risks—exactly what anyone initiating a project needs at the outset. It's the adult self who then harnesses the child's creative energy and brings it to fruition. Whether it's in the process of building a career, raising a family or growing vegetables, the adult finishes what the child within starts and by doing so, contributes to her world. Following through with her creativity is one way in which a woman expresses her adult identity.

With a strong adult in charge, you'll follow through to the completion of a project and trust that the inner warrior will take care of the child in the face of any possible external criticism or rejection. While defending the child within from any external negativity, the warrior must also combat the inner critic so that the child won't be paralyzed by self-doubt. Finishing any project brings satisfaction and reinforces your confidence in your ability to do it again.

If you're overweight, you may not be in touch with your creative energy. At some point, compulsive eating and obsessive thinking about food, weight, and dieting could have begun to monopolize most of your inner resources. You could have very little energy left inside with which to pursue creative activities. The lack of creative fulfillment in your life is a significant loss and it reinforces the feelings of boredom and emptiness that encourage overeating.

Everyone needs creative fulfillment for a meaningful existence. Love, work, and relationships aren't enough. You also need to feel like you're doing something constructive, productive, and rewarding in your life. Creativity can encompass anything from problem solving to scientific research; from architecture or engineering to cooking or gardening; from arts and crafts to building and construction. Business, marketing, and advertising are creative as well.

Engaging in creativity is fulfilling and empowering. You'll feel good about yourself when you accomplish something creative. This supports your self-esteem and the sense that you're living a full life. When you're creative, you see that you can make yourself happy. Creativity is also something you share with others. When you're expressing yourself freely, collaborating with like-minded individuals on a creative project or showing your work to an audience, you experience a sense of fulfillment that makes filling up with food completely unnecessary.

Being empowered also supports creativity. The process of facing, grieving, and letting go of the pain and hurt of your childhood will enable you to heal your wounds and reclaim your power. When you feel thus empowered, the fear of failing at creativity or being attacked by internal or external critics will disappear, and you'll then be able to take up the violin, enter design school, start your novel, or learn to dance.

When you feel empowered, failure isn't threatening. You can explore your creativity in any number of areas and whatever the outcome, you can be confident that the act of being creative is a reward in itself. Being empowered means knowing that you needn't be proficient at your creative pursuit right from the outset because if you stay with it, eventually you'll get the hang of it. You'll also understand the difference between commercial work and doing something simply for the fulfillment it brings. Florence doesn't have to make professional-quality drawings in the workshop (or on her own) in order for her creativity to be meaningful to her.

In fact, the commercial marketplace often has very little to do with artistic quality or creative vision. By engaging in a variety of creative modalities, Florence is overcoming the negativity of her inner critic as well as her fears of external criticism. Incidentally, Florence's piano playing is improving through her growth as an artist.

Florence has had such a vicious inner critic that sometimes it has interfered with her ability to perform, find employment, or even to establish intimate relationships. This extremely critical, paralyzing internalized parent is the "inner killer" because it destroys inspiration, initiative, and motivation and fosters hopelessness and despair.

Sadly, many people have a similar killer in their psyche and as soon as they get a burst of inspiration, it immediately begins to attack them. The inner killer is in agreement with external critics, and this combination is lethal to someone's nascent creativity. The solution to this is to "kill the killer." The visualization exercise in chapter 5, "Combating the Inner Opponent," is helpful in situations like this. It's empowering to imagine the warrior defending your creativity by eliminating the killer from the picture. It's a justifiable act of self-defense.

Being creative is truly filling. No amount of the most delicious food could ever compete with the deep and enduring gratification that comes from creative expression. Knowing that through creativity, you're able to meet your own needs and meaningfully connect to others, you can be less dependent on external sources of fulfillment, like food. When you know that you have the power to make yourself this happy and this full, while also making a contribution to the world, the allure of any addictive substance or activity will fade away.

8

CONSCIOUS EATING: EATING AS AN ADULT, NOT AS A CHILD

The child within you eats as a way to soothe her pain, stuff down anger, or fill an emotional void. An adult eats for nutrition and pleasure, but with moderation and restraint. Food is first and foremost *fuel* for your body. The primary reason an adult eats is to achieve and maintain an optimal state of health. Conscious eating is a matter of being the adult and eating for health, rather than allowing the child to be in charge, eating for emotional reasons.

When you're well nourished and eating a regular balanced diet, rich in all the necessary nutrients, you'll have fewer cravings for snacks and especially for junk food. If you eat as an adult and fill your body with good-quality, natural, whole foods, as opposed to processed, high-calorie, nutritionally depleted foods you'll feel satisfied and content. You'll be able to go on to the next thing you'd like to do, as opposed to feeling hungry, irritable, and still focused on food.

If the child is in charge of your eating, she'll be attracted to the wrong types of foods because she's looking for comfort and healing, not nutrition. She'll choose highly refined carbohydrates, high-fat, or highly seasoned food, all of which increase your cravings. Healthy eating encourages more of the same because the satisfaction and sense of well-being you experience after eating something nutritious create positive reinforcement. Child-driven dysfunctional eating backfires, because unhealthy food gives you neither the nutrition nor the emotional gratification you need, so you're never satisfied, no matter how much you eat.

Highly processed foods provide intense stimulation but little nutritional value. When we eat a lot of refined flour and sugar, high-fructose corn syrup, and saturated fat instead of fruits and vegetables, whole grains, and legumes, we're substituting intense flavor and texture for wholesome nutrition and putting our health at risk. The skyrocketing rates of obesity, diabetes, heart disease, and cancer aren't a coincidence. Study after study shows a correlation between our current diet and ill health.

We've gotten into some bad eating habits due to our busy lifestyles; an unconscious, cavalier attitude about nutrition; and the ubiquity of convenience foods. Our lives lack meaning and purpose and our relationships are unsatisfying. We spend too much time in front of computer screens and not enough time pursuing the things that will bring true happiness. The child within feels chronically unfulfilled and returns, over and over, to yummy food to meet her needs. Aside from dealing with our real needs and feelings, we'll have to get back to a more natural way of eating if we want to be healthy and break free of our cravings. This won't be easy for everyone. Many people are so used to eating bad quality food that they can't appreciate the flavors and textures of simple, healthy food. Such individuals will have to learn to enjoy healthy food choices.

If you're one of these people, you'll need to shift your diet away from processed foods and gradually introduce fresh, whole foods. This shift will "resensitize" your previously overstimulated palate, so that you come to appreciate natural flavors and textures. When your palate has been retrained to enjoy natural, whole foods, and you enjoy the experience of well-being that comes from eating right, your cravings for unhealthy food will subside.

THE EMOTIONAL BASIS OF FOOD CRAVINGS

Certain cravings relate to specific emotional states and needs. *Carbohydrate cravings,* for example, relate to feelings of emptiness and the need to feel full. If you stuff yourself with carbs, the emotional emptiness will be temporarily alleviated. Also, carbohydrates act as a natural calming agent. You'll be so drowsy after a big meal of pasta and garlic bread that your usual state of anxiety will be diminished. Refined carbohydrates, however, cause a rapid spike and then an equally rapid drop in blood glucose, which lead you to crave more of these.

When becoming conscious about your carbohydrate cravings, it's important that you look at why you're feeling empty inside, or why you need to avoid your issues by overstuffing yourself with food that makes you feel drowsy. As conscious adult, you'll understand that food will never compensate for your real needs. You'll begin to see that if you're in the habit of stuffing yourself with carbs, they can't ever make you feel full or sedated enough. In the absence of a strong adult, the child within will persevere in the hopes of obtaining healing, comfort, and fulfillment. Using carbs to avoid dealing with your emotional issues won't make these issues go away, so if the child is in charge, you'll have to continue carbo-loading to keep your needs and feelings at bay.

If you crave *rich, sweet, creamy foods* like cheese, ice cream, pudding, or custard, it could be linked to the first such food you ever had: mother's milk or formula. This was your first source of comfort and soothing. If you didn't experience enough reassurance or nurturing while growing up, it's likely that you weren't able to properly develop your own self-comforting and self-soothing mechanisms as an adult. For this reason, you may turn to comfort foods, which provide the child within with a false sense of soothing and reassurance. The truth is that the need for comfort is natural and persists throughout life, so you'll have to find a better way to comfort yourself or you'll never be free of this craving.

If you crave *chewy, crunchy foods,* you may be dealing with repressed anger. The acts of biting and chewing are associated with the most primitive survival instincts; a craving for foods you can sink your teeth into can represent unconscious aggression. If you take the time to sit with the child within and explore her feelings, you may discover this buried anger, and then you'll be able to deal directly with what this craving represents.

Becoming conscious around eating means not only looking at *what* you eat but at *how* you eat. Are you eating on the run, grabbing whatever is at hand and eating as you drive, walk or use public transportation? Are you eating standing up at the kitchen counter or in front of the TV? Do you eat while talking on the phone? All of these encourage distracted, unconscious eating where you're barely aware of what you're consuming. Instead, why don't you try making eating a deliberate act? Take a few minutes to sit at a table, pay attention to the food, and enjoy the experience of eating, rather than swallowing food down automatically.

Perhaps this is one reason why food is so oversaturated with intense, artificial flavors. If we're all eating with a minority of our attention paid to the food, it's no wonder manufacturers have to make it overstimulating. Distracted eating will encourage overeating for a few reasons: You don't notice how much you're consuming so you keep eating, unaware of what you've taken in. You can't enjoy the experience and may want to eat more in order to feel satisfied. Inattentive eating makes it hard to know when you're feeling full and the more you overfill your stomach, the more it stretches, encouraging further overeating.

If your attention isn't on what you're eating, the child within takes over and eats for her own, emotional reasons. If you begin paying attention to what you're eating, the adult will be in charge. You'll be able to have far greater enjoyment of smaller amounts of simpler food. Conscious eating is not reflex, automatic, or reactive eating, but is deliberate and aware. It's about being able to eat for the right reasons and truly savor what you're eating. As a result, you'll get more out of less.

It's not inevitable that you should be driven by the child within to succumb to your cravings or forced by the internalized parent to deny yourself enjoyment. Eating consciously is eating as an adult; it's eating in balance, enjoying the flavor, texture, and ceremony of your food and the health benefits of a good diet. If you're feeding your physical appetite and bodily requirements as opposed to the needs arising from your emotional wounds, you'll feel more full and satisfied with smaller portions of higher quality food.

OVERVALUED FOODS AND FREEDOM FROM ADDICTION

While my patient Billie has been trying to lose weight, the child within her has been playing this game. She's figured out that if she eats a few olives and a small amount of cheese in the evening, it will satisfy her cravings and keep her from having a binge. The problem is that she's now become obsessed with these olives and this bit of cheese and is compulsive in the use of this "solution" to her evening urges to overeat.

She's transferred her obsessive thinking and compulsive behavior from the ice cream she used to binge on to the olives and cheese that she now eats at night. The child within is still in charge, and Billie needs to see that she won't be free of her overeating problem until the adult takes over and food is no longer so immensely important to her.

Diet programs frequently say, "you can eat all the foods you love and still lose weight!" They're giving a mixed message here, saying that eating the foods you love will make you fat, but that you have to have them. They're implying that there's no way you'll be able to stay on the diet if you have to deprive yourself of your "favorite foods." Because weight loss (and not freedom) is the goal, the diet program appeals to the child within by helping her to cheat, so she can literally have her cake (or ice cream) and eat it too.

But why is it so important to keep eating certain (unhealthy, fattening) foods? The implication is that you can't be happy if they aren't in your life; these foods are crucial to your emotional survival, despite keeping you heavy and threatening your physical health. This problem is evident in the way that people have terrible trouble giving up their favorite foods. Even when they're diagnosed with diabetes, high cholesterol or high blood pressure and are advised to give up certain foods in order to prevent serious health problems, many people can't.

It's obvious that the child within is in charge here, refusing to let go of the foods that she's convinced she needs. Diet programs collude with the child within, telling her that she needn't be deprived. They offer "diet" substitutes for her favorite foods. The child within may be naive but she's not stupid and pretty quickly, she'll recognize that diet versions of her beloved brownies, ice cream, pizza, and lasagna can never live up to the real thing. She'll often compensate for her feelings of disappointment with these diet foods by eating them to excess.

The more processed and chemical-filled these diet versions are compared to the real favorite foods of the child within, the less healthy they are and the less satisfaction they give. The disappointment the child within feels over the diet foods will eventually undermine your weight-loss plan. It would be healthier to have an occasional piece of cake made with real-food ingredients, than regular servings of these nutritionally suspect "diet" foods.

If you're the rare person who's okay with substitute foods, you still don't win. You'll still be obsessed with your favorite foods and compelled to eat them, just in their diet versions. When you absolutely have to eat pizza or brownies because you can't live without them, it means that your cravings have gotten the best of you. This isn't freedom; it's enslavement to addiction. In order to be happy, you must let go of your intense, child-like attachment to certain foods and take the charge off eating, in general. This is accomplished first, by understanding the symbolic meaning of these "overvalued foods" to the child within. You'll have to face and grieve the unmet childhood needs that these overly important foods are meant to replace.

Then, you'll have to take steps to replace these favorite foods with what you really need today: the self-care you've been procrastinating about, the meaningful relationships you might have been avoiding, and the creative project that's sitting unfinished or the community work that you want to start. When you follow your dreams and pursue what your heart desires, the cravings of your taste buds will disappear.

Understanding the meaning of specific cravings is one way to overcome them. As I said, it has meaning if you crave sweets, fatty or crunchy foods, or carbs. A specific craving doesn't just mean that you like a particular food. It's about having a *psychological attachment* to the *symbolic meaning* of a certain food. This need to have a particular food is so strong that it becomes "pathological," in the diabetic who can't give up sweets or the hypertensive who can't stop eating salty foods.

If there are any foods that you can't give up, you'll need to get to the bottom of your attachment to them. Otherwise, there will be no peace for you as you try to heal your food addiction, change your eating habits, and improve your life. It's all about differentiating what the child within craves as opposed to what you as an adult truly want. The child within overvalues a particular food or group of foods because she's convinced that these foods will fix her problems. Why does a person become overly attached to a particular food? It's not completely clear.

Some scientists say that foods high in saturated fat, refined sugar, or processed flour can cause the release of endorphins, which are also released when people use chemical opiates such as heroin, Demerol, or codeine. They say that these foods mimic the "rush" a person feels on heroin or similar drugs. It may be that they oversaturate and thus desensitize the reward pathway in the brain, so that the brain craves more of these particular foods in the same physiological way as a person develops cravings for heroin, cocaine, or alcohol.

Is it necessary, then, to completely deprive yourself of the foods you love most? The answer is "no," because self-deprivation is the purview of the perfectionist internalized parent. Food is an important source of pleasure. If we allow the parent to take away our pleasure, life becomes dreary and the child within will rebel. An excess of anything, however, isn't healthy for you, emotionally or physically. As a conscious adult, you'll need to find a reasonable balance between what tastes good and what's good for you.

If you like sweets, you can eat healthier food than the chocolate or cookies you crave. In fact, if you eat more fresh fruit and less candy, your sugar cravings will decrease significantly, in part because of corresponding changes in the brain's reward pathway and in part because your blood sugar will stabilize. More importantly, if you crave sweets you can look at what these sweets *represent* to you. Are you feeling embittered? Do you need more sweetness in your life? If so, choose to have more real sweetness in the form of greater self-love, more meaningful relationships, or more creative fulfill-ment. In this way, the majority of sweetness will be present in the actual content of your life.

When it comes to sweets, for certain individuals only the most refined sug-ars will satisfy. This is because these individuals have what I call a "burnt-out palate." They're so used to eating extremely sweet food that often they can't appreciate or even taste less intense and more natural flavors. For these indi-viduals, a course of *palate rehabilitation* is required.

If you're used to eating an excess of refined sugar, vegetables will taste bit-ter and fresh fruit will seem bland. Gradually decreasing your sugar intake will enable you to begin enjoying simple, healthy food. Retraining the palate also applies to people who eat a lot of spicy, salty, fatty, or deep-fried foods.

Palate rehabilitation will resensitize your taste buds so that you can begin to enjoy healthy foods. The more fresh, wholesome food you eat, the more you'll recognize how good it feels to eat healthy and how bad your body feels when you don't. This is an important behavioral change, but it can't be a replace-ment for understanding and addressing the real reasons for your intense food cravings. Behavioral support is necessary in all cases of psychological change, but it isn't sufficient. The behavioral adjustments you make will only be effec-tive if they're combined with the work the adult self is doing in healing and nurturing the child within and giving her what she really craves.

Foods take on symbolic meaning because they're associated with the peo-ple, places, and moments of your life. You might have eaten certain foods as a child. Perhaps you were given milk and cookies when you were ill, or re-warded for a good grade with a chocolate bar. Perhaps you always had mashed potatoes at weekly family dinners. In this way, these foods become associated with feelings of security, comfort, or love.

After her parents got divorced, my patient Melinda always went out for ice cream with her father when he came to visit her on Sundays. Ice cream became associated with the feelings of happiness and belonging that Melinda experienced every time she saw her father. Now she unconsciously turns to ice cream every time she wants to reproduce the same feelings.

Perhaps you're someone who grew up with a mother who was not very demonstrative in her affection, but who always baked. You grew up with few hugs but lots of brownies, cakes, and pies. These desserts were the next best thing to the physical affection that was missing in your childhood, and they came to represent maternal love. For this reason, it would be hard for you to give them up. You'll need to discover the specific symbolism of the foods you crave in order to break the spell they have on you. If not, you'll forever be enchanted by the allure of these foods.

By working with the child within, you become empowered both to let go of overvalued foods and to continue with the work of healing and nurturing yourself. Every time you practice building the adult-child connection, you're taking responsibility for your own happiness and when you feel like happiness is within your power, your food cravings begin to disappear.

You don't become healthy or free by eating the "diet" versions of the foods you crave. It's just a way for the diet industry to keep you caught up in the (obsessive-compulsive) diet mentality. The industry profits from having dieters spend money on their programs, and by getting people to buy diet versions of their favorite foods. Aside from being unhealthy, diet foods promote addiction by playing right into the pathological hope of the child within.

Diet plans promise that you'll be able to "eat all the foods you love and still lose weight," the catch being that these foods must be the ones sold by that particular program. Once you let go of the child's obsessive belief in the power of these foods and her compulsive need to eat them, you'll see diet foods for the false solution that they are.

With the adult self in charge of your eating, you'll be able to let go of your pathological relationship with certain foods and with food, in general. You'll be free to eat good-tasting, healthy food in moderation, and the weight will come off, perhaps less quickly than the diets might promise you, but with far fewer negative psychological and physical health implications.

Diet companies take advantage of the child's unmet needs for healing and nurturing, as well as her pathological attachment to quick, easy, and false solutions. They may not be aware of the existence of the child within, but they understand that a big part of you wants things to be superficial, effortless, and instantaneous. In their willingness to exploit your child-like desire for the "quick fix" of deeper issues, they're only too happy to provide you with a way to cheat, in the form of diet foods. You don't have to go along with this, however. If you do the work as outlined in this book, you won't be taken in by the spurious promises of the diet industry.

My patient Melinda indulged the child within by succumbing to her cravings, first through eating regular ice cream, then turning to the diet version. Unfortunately, eating diet ice cream only reinforced her obsessive thoughts about this food and her compulsive behavior around eating it. Instead of breaking the spell that ice cream had over her, substituting the less-satisfying diet version for the real food only intensified Melinda's cravings.

The belief that you need to eat diet foods is supported by the internalized parent who says to the child within, "You're fat. You need to lose weight!" Even very thin women eat diet foods if they believe the internalized parent who tells them that they need to stay thin or become thinner.

The rigid, demanding internalized parent tells the child within that she mustn't eat her favorite, fattening foods. The diet companies seduce the child within when they give her an out by providing her with diet versions. As a fully fledged, empowered adult, you'll be able to silence the internalized parent so that the child doesn't have to react against it. The child within will come to trust your adult self to eat consciously, making diet food irrelevant.

Instead of it being such a charged subject, food needs to take its proper place in your psyche and your life. The adult in you will do this by healing the wounds that have caused you to overvalue food either in a positive way, where some foods are seen to be "good," or in a negative way where they're "bad."

With the child within in charge, you could overindulge in a comfort food like pasta, thinking it will make you feel better. If the child listens to the internalized parent, you could go on bizarre diets where you'll eat large amounts of "good" foods, like soup or grapefruit, or you'll stop eating bread or potatoes because you believe that "carbs are bad."

My patient Billie told a story about her young friend Peggy, who had to be treated in the emergency room after experiencing a dangerous heart arrhythmia. Blood tests done in the ER revealed that Peggy's potassium levels were abnormally low, and that this potassium deficiency was responsible for the irregular heartbeat. Later, when she was back at home, Peggy confessed to Billie that she'd stopped eating all fruits and vegetables because they had carbohydrates in them. As a result, she was getting nearly no potassium in her food. After months of doing this, she was dangerously malnourished. Placing such a negative value on carbohydrates caused Peggy to deplete her body of a necessary nutrient and nearly killed her.

Several years ago I went to school with a young woman named Phyllis. She avoided sugar but drank at least a dozen cans of diet soda a day. She was always full from the soda, so she ate very little healthy food. Her addiction to diet pop was undermining her health.

Letting go of food addiction has to include letting go of overvaluing (or vilifying) any specific type of food. Freedom from addiction is about not being overly invested in anything, whether it's a forbidden food, a favorite food, a favorite thing to drink or the thing you most love to buy. You're free from addiction when you don't have anything in your life that you feel you can't live without. It's having nothing in your life that you'd risk your health for. Freedom from addiction isn't about forcing yourself to do without something you desperately feel you need. Nor is it finding a potentially worse substitute for this thing. It's no longer being obsessed with a thing or activity or compelled to indulge in it. Freedom is possible and within your grasp, and becoming conscious is the first step.

What is consciousness? To me, it's waking up and seeing past the surfaces of things, right to the deepest layers. It's moving from a superficial awareness to an understanding of what's really going on within you and around you. It's no longer accepting that what you hear, see, or are told is the whole truth. Instead, it involves questioning the nature of things. Consciousness is about not merely accepting the status quo, but being skeptical about the messages you're receiving, whether from internal or external sources. It's questioning the motivations of those who are telling you things that seem too good to be true, and asking yourself whether they have your best interests or their own selfish needs at heart.

Consciousness is an adult function. Adult thinking is sophisticated and incisive, while a child's thinking is simple and concrete. Adults can see below the surface of things, but a child only sees what's directly in front of her. It's this part of you that gets fooled into thinking that "what you see is what you get." Adult consciousness around eating involves understanding the unconscious emotional wounds that drive you to eat in a certain way, the subtle societal factors that support this way of eating and the internal conflicts that promote your attitudes and behaviors around food. With consciousness, you'll have power to know yourself and to change.

Consciousness promotes change for the right reasons, because your motivation will be health and freedom from addiction, as opposed to trying to lose weight in order to please the inner critic. Working with the child within strengthens your experience of being an empowered adult around food, and feeling more empowered increases your motivation to eat for health and enjoyment, not for love or healing. Rather than being caught in the child-driven vicious circle of overeating, feeling shame and remorse, and then overeating to self-soothe, you'll enter a positive cycle of eating like an adult that, in turn, will reinforce your confidence regarding your ability to eat with consciousness.

Being conscious, you recognize that you have a real choice about what you eat and that you don't have to be a slave to whatever food or diet is "in" or "out" at any given time. For example, you'll be able to eat in a balanced way, making conscious choices about foods that you saw as "bad" in the recent past, like eggs, fats, or carbohydrates. You'll understand that none of these foods is necessarily "bad."

The diet industry likes to jump on the "food fad" bandwagon and vilify certain foods in order to sell you diet substitutes for the so-called bad foods. Consciousness enables you to see that you can eat many of these so-called bad foods in moderation, as long as they're in a healthy form. Eggs are an excellent source of low-calorie protein, and their association with high cholesterol in the body has yet to be conclusively demonstrated. Fats are needed to keep your blood sugar and appetite stable and good fats play a role in reducing inflammation associated with cancer and heart disease. Complex carbohydrates are essential for proper nutrition, and very low-carb diets have been shown to cause serious illness such as kidney disease; a result of too much protein being processed by these organs.

You'll recognize that the typical North American diet of today, despite the availability of an enormous variety of good-quality food, is extremely limited, lacking in imagination and not particularly healthy. North Americans eat an excess of red meat, processed sugar, flour and corn products, high-fat and deep-fried foods. We eat a minimum of vegetables and drink high-calorie soda pop, fruit drinks or juices instead of eating nutritious fruit. With consciousness, you'll be able to let go of your unhealthy eating habits and include a wider variety of wholesome foods in your daily diet.

Consciousness includes having an open mind and being curious about why things are a certain way. The conscious adult is never rigid or black-and-white in her thinking. She wants to know, so she pays close attention to what's really happening and to what she's being told. She won't be sold a bill of goods. The conscious adult examines the consequences that follow her choices and learns to anticipate what will result from certain decisions.

The child within engages in avoidance, denial, and "magical thinking." She ignores painful truths and convinces herself that things will be the way that she wants them to be. According to her, "this diet will make me lose weight quickly and easily," but reality ultimately catches up with this unrealistic form of thinking and sooner or later, the diet will fail.

The unconscious child within is seduced by things in pretty packages, regardless of whether they have any substance to them. Diet plans are extremely well marketed, with ecstatic testimonials from the few individuals who were able, at least temporarily, to lose weight by following the program. The conscious adult looks beyond the surface to what is driving her urge to overeat, and seeks to resolve her compulsive eating by addressing the root cause of it, rather than imposing a superficial solution.

Consciousness gives you power because it offers you more choices in how to act. For example, it enables you to understand the real source of your urge to overeat. You can tune in to your cravings and ask yourself what you're really hungry for. You can get in touch with the unmet needs and unhealed wounds of the child within and see that this emotional "unfinished business" is what's driving your compulsive eating.

Consciousness allows you to recognize the consequences of your dysfunctional eating behavior. For example, you might have thought that you could lose weight by skipping breakfast, but often, hunger will kick in and you end up eating a mid-morning donut. With consciousness, you'll recognize that without a nutritious breakfast, you feel light-headed and can't focus on your work. After you have the donut, the refined sugar and flour and deep-fried fat cause you to feel heavy, tired, and queasy. You might have experienced these same sensations in the past but in the absence of consciousness, you might not have associated them with your choice to skip breakfast and then opt for a donut. With consciousness, these sensations become clearly defined and connected to their source.

When you have only a vague feeling of malaise, you have no power to act differently. Becoming conscious about the food choices you just made will empower you in the future to eat a balanced breakfast before you leave for work.

Consciousness can change your binge-eating behavior. With consciousness, you can tune in to your genuine needs and feelings, and stop the binge as soon as you recognize that it's not what you really want. Prior to becoming conscious, the binge would be something that you did automatically and without thinking. Consciousness brings the child's needs to light. Once you're aware of them, you can deal with these needs directly, rather than by overeating.

At each stage of your developing consciousness, you'll have more choice. The more conscious you are, the sooner you'll be able to access the child within and choose to give her love, healing, and fulfillment instead of chips, chocolate, and ice cream. The more aware you become of your real needs, and the more you practice meeting them in a meaningful way, the less you'll want to binge.

Consciousness begins with the intention to face the truth. The good news is that once you set the intention, developing greater consciousness is something that takes on a life of its own. By this I mean that once you decide that you want to be more conscious about your eating (and everything else in your life), the work you do toward growing your awareness will be self-perpetuating. Consciousness breeds more consciousness. By asking questions, going beyond the surface of things and learning the truth, your happiness will grow and your suffering will diminish, all of which will motivate you to continue developing your consciousness.

EXERCISES FOR THE DEVELOPMENT OF CONSCIOUSNESS

If you're constantly busy and rushing around, you won't be able to develop your consciousness because it's something that needs time and space to grow. Quiet contemplation is the growing medium for consciousness, just as rich soil is needed to grow a fruit tree. Giving your consciousness time and space to grow will bear you the fruit of a happier, more empowered, and successful existence. Anyone can become more conscious if they make the time to do so.

THE BODY SCAN

This is a basic exercise that will help you become more conscious of your physical sensations and enable you to begin differentiating real hunger from emotional emptiness or neediness. All you have to do is find a quiet place to sit and begin to pay attention to all the parts of your body, one by one, inside and out.

Notice your feet on the ground and whether they feel heavy or light. Notice your legs and how they feel. Do they seem solid, weak, wobbly, or well grounded? Bring your attention to your torso, and notice what it feels like to be sitting on the chair. Do you feel settled in, or does it feel like you're hovering just above the chair? Notice your internal organs. Is your belly grumbling, tight, achy, or fluttery? Do you feel a sense of fullness or emptiness in your belly? Do you feel hunger, or is it just nervous energy in there?

Bring your attention up to your chest. Is there any pain or soreness in the muscles of your chest? Can you feel your heart beating? Is it slow and steady or is your pulse throbbing or racing? Notice your breathing and what's happening as you inhale and exhale. Does the breath get stuck at the top of your lungs, or does it fill your lungs all the way to the bottom of your diaphragm?

Notice your neck and shoulders and whether there's any tightness there. Does your neck feel loose and free, or sore and restricted? Do you have a lump in your throat or is your swallowing easy? Notice your face and if any muscles are clenched in your jaw, mouth, or cheeks or around your eyes. Notice if your throat is dry or sore, if there's any ringing in your ears or twitching in your eyelid. Finally, notice if your body in general feels calm or jumpy. Are your muscles relaxed or restless?

Paying this type of close attention to your body and its sensations allows you to know yourself in a deeper way than ever before. If you do this now and then, you'll become familiar with your body's rhythms and needs. You'll learn to differentiate physical hunger from anxiety, boredom, loneliness, or pain. Your eating will become responsive to what's really happening in your body, not to your emotional needs.

The Emotional Check In

This is an exercise for getting in touch with your feelings. All you have to do is take a moment out of your busy life to tune in to what's going on with you emotionally. Maybe you're having a physical sensation of discomfort that hints of a feeling underneath. Put your attention on this sensation, and see whether the feeling emerges into consciousness.

Maybe you're feeling anxious or agitated. Perhaps you're nervous or about something specific, but maybe there's another emotion lurking beneath the surface. Bring your attention to this restless feeling and you might find that there's sadness, loneliness, anger, or some other emotion lying just below the superficial experience of anxiety.

When you practice tuning in to your emotions, it makes you more adept at identifying what you're feeling at any moment. When connecting to your feelings, don't try to analyze your experience; this will take you out of your feelings and into your thoughts. It's a lot easier to access your emotions when you're not trying to "figure out" what's going on inside you.

If you get in touch with sadness, for example, and you don't understand why you're feeling sad right now, you don't need to have an immediate answer. Just paying attention to your emotions will help you be more conscious of what's going on inside you, and when the child within is ready, she'll offer up some insights about why you happen to be sad.

Accessing your emotions gives you a greater awareness of yourself. When you know what you feel, you can know what you want. In turn, knowing what you want enables you to know what to do. Emotions lead to desires, and desires lead to actions. Conscious choice and conscious behavior stem from consciousness about your true emotions and your true needs.

Conquering the Urge

Here's an exercise to help develop your consciousness with regard to food cravings. When you're experiencing a powerful urge to eat that you know isn't from hunger (let's say it's after dinner, and you've had all the fuel you need for the day), here's something you can do to overcome the urge to eat compulsively.

First, notice the urge within you. To an unconscious, needy child this urge feels overwhelming but to the conscious adult, it's just a feeling. A child feels small and powerless in the face of her food cravings, but a conscious adult knows that she's stronger than any urge.

In the past, you might have succumbed to the urge to eat at this point. Instead, just observe as the urge intensifies. The child within might be screaming, "I have to eat something right now!" The adult, however, knows that nothing bad will happen if she doesn't give in to the urge, and she simply continues to observe it. At the same time, knowing what it is the child really needs, you can give the child some loving attention and reassure her that she's going to be okay.

Eventually, the urge to eat will peak. (Often this happens after only a few minutes.) At its worst, you see that the urge is really not so bad. It's not an unbearable pain or a real physical need. In fact, there's no physical component to it whatsoever. The child is convinced that she must give in to the urge, but the adult can see that the child is mistaken. Resisting the urge has caused nothing bad to happen.

Finally, the urge begins to wane. Notice that you were able to resist it, even at its strongest. Having resisted the temptation to overeat, you can see that you're stronger than the urge, and the adult can tell the child within that she needn't be overwhelmed by her urges again. The adult is clearly more powerful than they are.

Not giving in to the urge enables you to gain a sense of mastery over it. Each time you do this exercise, you'll see that not only is the urge far less powerful than you thought it was, but you're able to resist it with less and less effort. The more you practice resisting the urge, the less intense each successive urge will be and the more infrequently they'll arise. Your consciousness about food cravings enables you to resist them, and in resisting your food cravings, your conscious understanding and mastery of them grows.

As you develop greater consciousness, you'll also have an increased awareness of the messages society is sending you about food and eating. This will enable you to identify all the contradictions that you encounter on a daily basis that make your relationship to food and eating more fraught and confusing than it ought to be. You'll be able to see that it's not your fault that you feel torn about whether to eat something when within a few pages of a woman's magazine there's a recipe for a rich dessert and then an article on the latest way to lose weight. With consciousness, you'll recognize that you live in a society that's giving mixed messages by focusing intensely on food and eating while at the same time strongly promoting dieting and thinness.

Consciousness will enable you to understand why delicacies like truffles, caviar, and foie gras are almost worshiped by certain members of our society, while at the same time things like salt, fat, and carbs are shunned as "evil." It will help you understand why we both idolize celebrity chefs and vilify people who take "too much" pleasure in eating, as though these folks are morally deficient and overly self-indulgent. We're a society obsessed with food and deeply conflicted about it. So many North Americans have narrowly, restricted, poor-quality diets, despite the huge variety of excellent food available to them. Too many people don't have enough to eat, and others deprive themselves unnecessarily out of the fear of gaining an ounce.

In the media, there's far too much emphasis on food, both positive and negative. It's an enormously charged subject. Our culture is as wounded around food as its individual members are, and this is a major factor in the current obesity epidemic. Becoming conscious will help you to let go of your confusion and learn to trust your own physical and emotional needs with regard to food and eating. You don't have to be a casualty of our society's craziness about food.

Consciousness will give you the clarity to see that because food is the only addictive substance that you need for your survival, your relationship to food will always be different from your relationship to anything else. Because you must eat several times a day, you can't abstain from food as you can from drugs or alcohol. In a sense, you're lucky that overeating is your addiction because it forces you to face the real issues underlying your problem.

You can't ignore food. You need it every day. Even if you fast, or go on a liquid diet for several weeks, you'll have to go back to eating solid food. Eventually, you'll have to deal with your disordered eating. A food addiction is a blessing in disguise. Having to eat on a regular basis gives you the perfect opportunity to become conscious about food.

You can choose to look at what you're eating and why you're eating it. You can get to the bottom of the problem, once and for all. If you're overweight, it becomes hard to deny that you have a problem, given your expanding waistline, sore knees, or shortness of breath. It's pretty hard to ignore food or deny your weight. If you choose to tune in to the real cause of the problem, instead of doing the endless cycle of dieting, you'll have a real chance, not only of losing the weight, but of being healed.

If you're awake and aware, you'll see the truth about the proliferation of food images bombarding you every day on TV, online, in magazines, and in restaurant windows. These images are representations of society's wounded, dysfunctional obsession with food. The media barrage you with information about the obesity epidemic, yet enormous plates of food are being served in restaurants and at fast food chains. Meanwhile, just down the street from the restaurant serving giant portions, people are lining up at the food bank.

An acquaintance of mine recently described her horror while driving by a local family-style restaurant that was advertising a special for a one-person meal consisting of a *32 ounce steak*. They were implying that eating two pounds of meat at one sitting should be desirable, when in fact an appropriate serving is about four ounces. I've seen ads for an ice-cream chain that sells a sundae with 15 scoops of ice cream. The other day, a local seafood chain was on TV promoting a four-course dinner including a creamy soup, a salad, rolls, a main course including pasta and a large dessert. At the same time as these restaurants are promoting their specials, politicians are promoting the newest antiobesity measures and the Internet is flashing pictures of latest celebrities who've lost weight. Local food programming showcases restaurants that serve outrageously sized mega-meals, while at the same time famous butter-loving chefs are either losing hundreds of pounds or being diagnosed with type 2 (obesity-related) diabetes.

There's a lot of attention on the epidemic of overweight children in North America, their soda-pop and French fries diet and their sedentary lifestyle. Also in the news lately are stories of ever more skinny fashion models, literally dropping dead from food restriction. Just recently, I learned that the gap between the weight of the average woman and the weight of the average model has gone from 8 percent in the 1990s to 23 percent today. The fashion runways are walked by shockingly skeletal teenagers, while the malls are walked by frighteningly overweight moms. Diet pill commercials compete with snack food ads for airtime, so it's no wonder that we feel confused. Consciousness will help you see that this type of bizarre split is really a battle between the *parent* and the *child* within our society.

The more repressive the "parents" in society are in preaching thinness and restrictive eating habits, the more the child within will go to one of two extremes: either she'll comply and starve herself or she'll defy the parent and see giant portions as desirable. The more the parent-figures in society try to force you to be "good," around eating and the more the fast-food outlets and cooking shows promote extreme overindulgence, the more the child within each of us will react either by dieting obsessively or by overeating.

With consciousness, you can see that you live in a consumer society that's driven by the childlike need to have "more" of everything, including food, in order to fill the emptiness within. However, as it promotes *having* more, it also shames you for *wanting* more. The parental elements of society, like our TV doctors, "diet gurus" and celebrity personal trainers who preach rigid adherence to strict diet and exercise plans are not giving the child within a viable alternative to overconsuming. They're actually making her want to overeat in reaction against these rules. The child cries, "I want more!" and the parent responds, "if you were a good child, you'd want less and you'd take less." This battle has been raging for a long time, and without consciousness, it will continue to do so.

Those who have an obedient child within may think that they're better off than those who have a rebellious child driving their eating behavior. Not so. It's the "good" child within who is thin but constantly obsessed with food and weight; she's the one who ends up in the hospital weighing 65 pounds due to anorexia nervosa. She's so good that she'll die trying to please the unreasonable parent in her psyche and in society.

Waking up and becoming more conscious will show you that taking a balanced approach is a wiser alternative to being in a child-parent war within your psyche or in society. Trying to please or spite the parent is for children. Healthy, conscious eating is an adult choice. Rather than letting the internalized or societal parent push the child around regarding food and weight, you can opt out of the craziness and just take loving care of your body and your health. You can enjoy food without being overly invested in what you eat and you can put your attention on the other important things in life aside from food and weight.

Consciousness also means that you hate neither your body because it isn't "thin enough" nor yourself because you can't achieve some unrealistic weight or shape. It means accepting and loving your body as it is now while dealing with what's driving your compulsive eating and weight problem. Consciousness involves understanding that you have a certain natural body type, and that trying to force yourself to become a smaller size is both physically and emotionally damaging to you. It means ruthlessly pursuing the deepest truth about your addiction(s), as well as dealing compassionately with yourself when you learn this truth. Ruthless compassion goes hand-in-hand with adult consciousness, and with it, you'll be empowered to choose a better way of dealing with food and weight.

Developing consciousness goes along with developing the adult self. You become conscious when you spend time deliberately working on being the adult, questioning your perceptions, feelings, beliefs, and expectations, and challenging your self-image and worldview as well as the way others look at you. Children are credulous; they believe everything they're told. An adult can question what she's being told. Consciousness means not swallowing every story that you hear, whether from an outer opponent or from the internalized parent.

Initially, it might be difficult to develop consciousness. It's not your fault. Our society supports an unquestioning, apathetic mind. It can be painful to be more conscious because you'll recognize your suffering and that of others, as well as all the injustices in life. Still, knowing the truth gives you the chance to take concrete action for the purposes of alleviating your own suffering and that of others. With your head in the sand of unconsciousness, you can't remedy any bad situation or recognize how unhappy or unfulfilled you might be. Nothing will change for the better if you remain unconscious, and it could easily get worse.

In general, despite some initial pain caused by finally facing some truths you've been avoiding, life will be so much better, richer, and easier with greater consciousness. With consciousness you feel more, but suffer less, because you're dealing with things as they really are rather than how the child wishes them to be. This will help you to avoid the nasty surprises and disappointments that come from having your illusions smashed.

The child within becomes angry and frustrated when she doesn't feel "in control" of things. In her helplessness, the child believes that control will compensate for her lack of power. The conscious adult, however, doesn't need to force people or situations to be any particular way. Rather than trying to be in control, she trusts herself to take good care of herself, and to deal with challenges in a realistic manner. This prevents a lot of unnecessary suffering.

Being conscious means being a warrior in life instead of a victim. This isn't an aggressive stance, but an empowered way of living in which you take responsibility for your life, so that you don't blame others for your present-day problems. Consciousness gives you the power to change your life for the better. It also enables you to experience yourself as a responsible, interdependent member of a greater whole.

Consciousness is more powerful than knowledge. In fact, it's what enables you to use your knowledge and understanding in order to affect positive change. A young woman named Louise was attending my overeater's workshop a few years ago and we were having a discussion about nutrition. She said, "I could give this talk. I know everything there is to know about healthy eating." Then, several of the other members chimed in. All these women knew exactly what they should be eating for optimal health. They possibly knew more than I did. The problem was that they couldn't bridge the gap between their adult awareness of proper nutrition and the compulsion of the child within to overeat.

There's ample information available these days about how to eat well, and yet Louise and many others still eat for comfort, soothing, fulfillment, or to bury unwanted feelings. The question is how can you go from someone who eats as a child to someone who eats as an adult? The answer begins with becoming more conscious.

Once you've become conscious of the child within and her unhealed wounds and unmet needs, you're well on your way toward overcoming compulsive eating. With conscious awareness of the inner conflict between the child within and the internalized parent, and the recognition of the need to be the empowered adult in your life, you can begin to follow the four-pronged approach outlined in this book: (1) facing the truth about your past, grieving your losses, and letting go of your wounds; (2) loving, affirming, and protecting the child within; (3) pursuing the things in life that will bring you true meaning and fulfillment; and (4) identifying and rejecting the negative messages of the inner and outer opponents. This work will bring the adult to the forefront of your psyche so it can be in charge of your eating and nutrition.

If you've been eating unconsciously out of apathy, ignorance, or inertia, or if you've just been eating in the way that your parents showed you, it's not too late to become conscious and empowered. I'll say it again: everything good requires work and time. The child within wants the quickest, easiest answer, but the adult in you knows that taking time to become conscious about what you eat will make you feel better, not just physically but in your entire being.

Eating isn't a neutral act. Everything you put in your mouth originated somewhere and was produced by someone. Consciousness around eating also means considering where food comes from, in addition to its nutritional value. A number of years ago, Frances Moore Lappe wrote a magnificent little book titled *Diet for a Small Planet*. I highly recommend it as a primer on conscious eating. The author was ahead of her time, and many of the things she was saying back then are being proven true today.

Her message is that there are limited resources in the world and we need to rethink how we grow, process, and distribute food. I share her belief that fewer people on the planet would be suffering from hunger or malnutrition if there were more consciousness and social responsibility on the part of the producers, distributors, and consumers of food.

For example, beef cattle require enormous amounts of water and land mass to raise them to maturity. We can grow 40,000 pounds of potatoes on one acre of land but only 250 pounds of beef. Today, the total livestock in the

United States outnumber the human population by a factor of 4 to 1, requiring vast amounts of land, water, energy, and other resources. Thinking about the ramifications of this can help you make conscious, responsible decisions about what you choose to eat. It's not just the taste or the nutritional value of food that we need to consider. We also need to think about what it means for each person on the planet to eat consciously and responsibly.

Certain countries have more lax standards when it comes to the spraying of pesticides or the use of growth hormones in animal production. These substances speed up the process of getting food to the consumer and lead to greater milk or meat production. Growth hormones used in the United States cause cows to have horribly swollen udders and other serious physical problems. The cows suffer terribly from the use of these hormones, but are we thinking about the suffering that's being caused to produce this milk, or how drinking milk produced with growth hormones could affect our developing children?

Pesticides are sprayed on crops all over the world, and although here in North America, there are bans on certain, extremely toxic sprays, the ones commonly used are still of concern. Compared to the general population, there are higher rates of cancer amongst the people who work in fields where these chemicals are sprayed and their children have a higher risk of illnesses such as leukemia.[1] If we eat this food, not only are we risking our own health but we're complicit in the suffering of others.

Years ago, a farm worker and organizer named Cesar Chavez organized a boycott of California grapes for the same reason. The boycott put pressure on the grape growers by affecting their bottom line, and the pesticides used on these farms were eventually replaced with less toxic ones. Cesar Chavez was a true hero, and it's too bad that few people remember his name today. His efforts not only helped the workers he was associated with, but they helped us all to have access to safer and more nutritious food.

Washing fruits or vegetables grown with pesticides, even with soap and water, doesn't eliminate the toxins that the plants have soaked up. Over time, farm animals fed with pesticide-treated grains accumulate high doses of them in their tissues. The higher up on the food chain they are, the greater a pesticide load they carry when they finally are processed for our kitchen tables. I believe that our increased rates of cancer are in part, related to these poisons being so pervasive in our foods.

Some pesticides act as hormone disrupters, potentially causing a number of serious medical conditions. Pesticides in the fields leach into the water table and spread to larger bodies of water, getting into the local fish and into the water given to the animals in the community. Eating animals raised on feed and water that contain pesticide residues gives us a double dose of these toxic substances.

The main objection I hear from people who choose not to eat organic food is that it's "too expensive." I think that this is a short-sighted way of looking at things. If more and more of us demanded a greater variety of organic food at the local grocery store, more farmers would begin farming organically and the prices would go down. Other people complain about the inferior quality of organic produce, saying that the fruit and vegetables are "uglier" and have more marks on them. Again, if more people insisted on stores stocking organic produce, more would be produced and stores would have a better selection of fruits and vegetables to sell.

If you eat foods that are lower in toxins, you're likely to live longer and have fewer medical problems. You'll spend less money on health insurance and medical care and have fewer sick days. All this will increase your earning potential and improve your quality of life. Saving money now by not buying organic food is shortchanging yourself because eating organic will pay off in the long run. By avoiding foods that are "too expensive" you're risking your own health, that of your loved ones, and that of the planet, all for the sake of a few dollars saved here and there.

It's my opinion that organic food is better for the planet. It conserves resources, decreases the overall toxin load, replenishes the soil, and preserves near-extinct varieties of fruits and vegetables. Animals raised organically are free of pesticide residues, hormones, and antibiotics, and have better-quality feed. Being allowed to roam free, they have better lives and therefore their tissues aren't filled with the stress hormones that we would then ingest. They're living creatures that deserve our compassion and respect. If we eat these animals, use their eggs, or drink their milk, the least we can do is care about the lives they're living.

We can trust that eating organic foods will not only keep us healthy, but it can help protect our fragile ecosystem. Conscious eating is global eating. It's going beyond the local grocery store or farmer's market and asking the important questions about where our food comes from and how it was made.

When a Therapist Is Necessary

A few years ago, my patient Lucinda shared with me that she had undermined a romantic relationship with a very nice young man because she couldn't believe that he could love her the way he professed. She unconsciously believed that everyone would reject of her, as her parents had done, and she was convinced that even her boyfriend couldn't really care for her the way he said he did.

According to her skewed view of the world, people would only want to use her or be contemptuous toward her, like her parents were. Through therapy, she was able to see that the young man had genuinely cared about her, and that there would be others who'd care in the future. Her view of relationships gradually began to more closely approximate reality, as her therapy enabled her to let go of some erroneous expectations.

The goal of my work is to help people to become more conscious, happier, and more successful. This means that they'll be able to see the truth about themselves and their lives, rather than allowing their fears or false beliefs to tell them how things are. Many people today are living like Lucinda, with a somewhat skewed version of reality based on the child's projections of her past experiences onto the present-day world.

Therapy can enable you to become more conscious and have a more realistic view of yourself, others, and the world. Another patient, Cassandra, recently told me that she had always thought that she was a very "nice" person, whose nature was to be there for others. After doing therapy for a while, she realized that she'd been conditioned by her parents to be a care-taker and that her true personality was a lot more independent and a lot less ingratiating.

She came to see that her emotional wounds had made her deviate from her authentic self. Through therapy, she learned the truth about the powerful woman she really is, and saw how her parents had failed her. Today, Cassandra literally laughs with glee when thinking about the new, genuine person she's discovered beneath the facade of her old, overly helpful persona.

In dealing with overeating and being overweight, therapy can be extremely beneficial. It's very tempting to unconsciously continue to use food as the way to meet the needs of the child within, rather than seeing it as enjoyable nutrition and finding more valid solutions to your emotional needs. If you're only a few pounds overweight or if you've never really struggled to lose weight, it's probable that your wounds aren't that deep or food isn't your primary addiction. In that case, this book and the exercises contained within should be enough to help you to understand and begin dealing with this problem.

If, however, you've been unhappily overweight for years, you'd probably benefit from the support of a trained psychotherapist, especially if you've never been able to lose weight or have dieted and then regained weight many times. Therapy could also help you change other behaviors; for example, a chronic habit of bad relationships, self-destructive or defeatist patterns of behavior, a long-term lack of confidence or self-esteem, or blocks in your creativity or career. If you experience difficulties with intimacy, chronic feelings of emptiness, despair, or anxiety, therapy could benefit you, as well.

A psychotherapist is someone who uses talking and listening as her therapeutic tools in order to help you to make positive changes in your beliefs, attitudes, and behaviors, and to break counterproductive patterns of thinking, feeling, or acting. She can assist you in building your self-esteem, developing your creativity, improving your relationships, fulfilling your potential, and healing your addictions.

A therapist is necessary when your problems aren't limited to overeating and being overweight. You may be someone who, as well as being overweight, also suffers from anxiety, depression, phobias, sleep disturbances, or a tendency to be impulsive or self-destructive. These problems could have arisen at the same time as the eating and weight problems or could be related to overeating and being overweight.

Some people overeat and gain weight in order to deal with their anxiety or depression, and some become anxious or depressed as a result of being addicted to food and being overweight. You might be someone who suffers from anxiety, lying awake at night, worrying about things. You could have gotten into the habit of nocturnal eating to calm your nerves. Conversely, your excessive eating and weight could be causing emotional or physical problems that interfere with your ability to sleep. A therapist can help you understand your issues and deal with them, whether they're the cause or the effect of your dysfunctional eating.

A therapist is also important in the maintenance of a healthy attitude and lifestyle. It's easy to get side-tracked around eating and weight. There are so many ways for the child within to get overwhelmed, and to want to act out or to give up. Even someone who's done a lot of healing can use the ongoing support of a therapist to help her stay conscious and empowered. It takes a fair amount of time to consolidate internal change, and as you're getting used to seeing yourself and dealing with things in a whole new way, therapy could help to remind you of what you've chosen, and why.

In my opinion, if more people engaged in good, constructive psychotherapy, the world would be a better place. Imagine how things would be if people were to get over their child-driven preoccupation with exploiting the world's resources in order to accumulate food, money, or power and instead learned how to truly love and to care about themselves, others, and the planet. Imagine therapy enabling more people to become conscious about the problems within them and around them.

Through therapy, we could see that we're all interconnected, and we could start to take responsibility for the part we play in the world, individually and as a society. We could live to pursue our real dreams and contribute to the betterment of our community and our world, rather than constantly compensating for what the child within never received while growing up. Psychotherapy could transform wounded, alienated child-centered individuals into happy, confident adults who make a positive contribution to society. Perhaps not everyone is amenable to treatment or able to change, but many people today could be helped with therapy, and in turn, could have more to offer to their loved ones and to the world, once they were healed and whole.

I sometimes call the work that I do "soul work," because I believe that if you're deeply wounded, you've become alienated from your true nature. If you're living with false beliefs about yourself and the world, if you feel helpless or out of control in your life, and if you're unable to live as your optimal self, then your soul is in need of healing. When therapy helps you to take responsibility for your problems, rediscover your true nature, heal your wounds, and own your power, it's also helping you to heal your soul.

My patients recognize that soul work is indeed what's happening, because when everything starts to come together in therapy, they experience a sense of wholeness that's greater than the symptom relief they've sought. The feeling within them of personal integration is more than can be accounted for by the separate problems that they've been resolving.

The soul, to me, is the essence of your being. It's your core, and it stores the basic energy that connects you to all other living creatures. The soul can be damaged by neglect, trauma, and brutality in childhood; it can be deeply bruised and, sadly, it can even be destroyed.

A sociopath is someone with a broken soul due to childhood trauma (or, perhaps, his or her genetic makeup). They're incapable of empathy or remorse, and are unable to take responsibility for their actions. They have no conscience and no motivation to change, as they blame everyone else for their problems. These individuals aren't appropriate candidates for psychotherapy, as they're unable to form the necessary "therapeutic alliance." They're most likely to be deceitful and manipulative toward the therapist and to resist any real change.

On the other hand, someone with a bruised or damaged soul can benefit a lot from therapy. Even when people don't realize that it's their soul that's wounded, or when those who help them don't understand that they're actually healing souls, soul work can happen. When healers practice ruthless compassion; when they pursue the truth relentlessly, with an attitude of loving kindness, patience, and understanding, souls can be healed and lives transformed.

I think that today, the soul of our communities and in fact, the soul of North America, is in crisis. It's evident in the rampant greed, rudeness, selfishness, addiction, competitiveness, aggression, materialism, and perversion. I'm not talking about a religious understanding of the soul, but the understanding that we've lost our way and we're suffering, and the world is suffering as a result. Therapy can awaken people to self-love and enable them to heal. As they're filled with positive self-regard, this will overflow to others and into their community.

Real love isn't given in the hope of receiving something in return but from the experience of emotional fullness. When you truly love the child within and feel fulfilled within yourself, it's then that you'll have the most to give. This is what real generosity springs from: the overflow of self-love. Self-love isn't the same as selfishness. Selfishness or self-centeredness is the result of the wounded child being in charge, pursuing healing through compulsively consuming food, resources, and other people. Self-love is the experience of being full and fulfilled, with love to share.

Good therapy can help transform wounded individuals with bruised souls into loving, generous people who have much more to give to themselves and to others. My goals in therapy are the following: to decrease the suffering you cause yourself, to decrease the suffering you cause others, to decrease the suffering you allow other to cause you, and to be free to express your authentic, optimal self. By loving the child within in a meaningful way and by deeply healing your soul, all these things will happen. You'll finally be free of addiction, free to pursue your true dreams, and empowered to share the best of yourself with the world.

NOTES

CHAPTER ONE: COMPULSIVE EATING

1. Nelson Bryce, "The Addictive Personality: Common Traits are Found," *New York Times,* January 18, 1983.

2. David J. Linden, *The Compass of Pleasure* (Viking Press, 2011).

3. Vincent J. Felitti, "Ursprunge des Suchtverhaltens—Evidenzen au seiner Studie zu belastenden Kindheitserfahrungen" ["The Origins of Addiction: Evidence from the Adverse Childhood Experiences Study"]. *Praxis der Kinderpsychologie und Kinderpsychiatrie* 52 (2003): 547–59.

4. Ibid., p. 8.

5. Vincent J. Felitti, Kathy Jakstis, Victoria Pepper, and Albert Ray, "Obesity: Problem, Solution or Both?" *The Permanente Journal* 14, no. 1 (2010): 24–30.

6. Traci Mann, A. Janet Tomiyama, Erika Westling, Ann-Marie Lew, Barbara Samuels, and Jason Chapman, "Medicare's Search for Effective Obesity Treatments: Diets Are Not the Answer," *American Psychologist* 62, no. 3 (2007): 220–33.

7. Ibid., p. 230.

CHAPTER SIX: A NEW YOU EMERGING

1. David J. Linden, "Addictive Personality? You Might Be a Leader," *New York Times,* July 23, 2011.

2. Eric J. Nestler and Robert C. Malenka, "The Addicted Brain," *Scientific American,* March 2004, 78–85.

CHAPTER EIGHT: CONSCIOUS EATING

1. K.L. Bassil, Catherine Vakil, M. Sanborn, D.C. Cole, J.S. Kaur, and K.J. Kerr, "Cancer Health Effects of Pesticides: Systematic Review," *Canadian Family Physician* 53, no. 10 (2007): 1704–11.

BIBLIOGRAPHY

Allan, Michael G., Ivers, Noah, and Sharma, Arya M. "Diets for Weight Loss and Prevention of Negative Health Outcomes." *Canadian Family Physician* 57, no. 8 (2011): 894–95.

Anda, Robert F., Felitti, Vincent J., Bremner, J. Douglas, Walker, John D., Whitfield, Charles, Perry, Bruce D., Dube, Shanta R., and Giles, Wayne H. "The Enduring Effects of Abuse and Related Adverse Experiences in Childhood: A Convergence of Evidence from Neurobiology and Epidemiology." *European Archives of Psychiatry and Clinical Neurosciences* 256 (2006): 174–86.

Bassil, K.L., Vakil, C., Sanborn, M., Cole, D.C., Kaur, J.S., and Kerr, K.J. "Cancer Health Effects of Pesticides: Systematic Review." *Canadian Family Physician* 53, no. 10 (2007): 1704–11.

Dube, Shanta R., Felitti, Vincent J., Dong, Maxia, Chapman, Daniel P., Giles, Wayne H., and Anda, Robert F. "Childhood Abuse, Neglect, and Household Dysfunction and the Risk of Illicit Drug Use: The Adverse Childhood Experiences Study." *Pediatrics* 111, no. 3 (2003): 564–72.

Dyson, Lowell K. "American Cuisine in the 20th Century: A Century of Change in America's Eating Patterns." *FoodReview* 2, no. 1 (2000): 2–8.

Epel, E.S., McEwen, B., Seeman, T., Matthews, K., Castellazzo, G., Brownell, K.D., Bell, J., and Ickovics, J.R. "Stress and Body Shape: Stress-induced Cortisol Secretion Is Consistently Greater among Women with Central Fat." *Psychosomatic Medicine* 62, no. 5 (2000): 623–32.

Felitti, Vincent J. "Ursprunge des Suchtverhaltens—Evidenzen au seiner Studie zu belastenden Kindsheitserfahrungen" ["The Origins of Addiction: Evidence from the Adverse Childhood Experiences Study"]. *Praxis der Kinderpsychologie und Kinderpsychiatrie* 52 (2003): 547–59.

Felitti, Vincent J., and Anda, Robert A. "The Relationship of Adverse Childhood Experiences to Adult Medical Disease, Psychiatric Disorders and Sexual Behavior: Implications for Healthcare." In *The Impact of Early Life Trauma on Health and Disease: The Hidden Epidemic,* ed. Ruth A. Lanius, Eric Vermetten, and Clair Pain, 77–87. Cambridge: Cambridge University Press, 2010.

Felitti, Vincent J., Jakstis, Kathy, Pepper, Victoria, and Ray, Albert. "Obesity: Problem, Solution, or Both?" *The Permanente Journal* 14, no. 1 (2010): 24–30.

Felitti, Vincent J., and Williams, Seleda A. "Long-Term Follow-Up and Analysis of More Than 100 Patients Who Each Lost More Than 100 Pounds." *The Permanente Journal* 2, no 3 (1998): 1–9.

Gilden Tsai, Adam, and Wadden, Thomas A. "Systematic Review: An Evaluation of Major Commercial Weight Loss Programs in the United States." *Annals of Internal Medicine* 142, no. 1 (2005): 56–66.

Grucza, Richard A., Krueger, Robert F., Racette, Susan B., Norberg, Karen E., Hipp, Pamela R., and Bierut, Laura J. "The Emerging Link between Alcoholism Risk and Obesity in the United States." *Archives of General Psychiatry* 67, no. 12 (2010): 1301–08.

Lappe, Frances Moore. *Diet for a Small Planet (20th Anniversary Edition).* New York: Ballantine Books, 1991.

Mann, Traci, Tomiyama, A. Janet, Westling, Erika, Lew, Ann-Marie, Samuels, Barbara, and Chapman, Jason. "Medicare's Search for Effective Obesity Treatments: Diets Are Not the Answer." *American Psychologist* 62, no. 3 (2007): 220–33.

Mentzer Morrison, Rosanna, Buzby, Jean C., and Hodan, Farah Wells. "Guess Who's Turning 100? Tracking a Century of American Eating." *Amber Waves.* US Department of Agriculture Economic Research Service, March 2010.

Nelson, Bryce. "The Addictive Personality: Common Traits Are Found." *The New York Times,* January 18, 1983.

Nestler, Eric J., and Malenka, Robert C. "The Addicted Brain." *Scientific American,* March 2004, pp. 78–85.

Peeke, P.M., and Chrousos, G.P. "Hypercortisolism and Obesity." *Annals of the New York Academy of Sciences* 771 (1995): 665–76.

Pollan, Michael. *In Defense of Food: An Eater's Manifesto.* New York: Penguin Books, 2008.

Rabin, Roni Caryn. "Can You Be Addicted to Foods?" *The New York Times,* January 5, 2011.

Sumithran, Priya, Prendergast, Luke A., Delbridge, Elizabeth, Purcell, Katrina, Shulkes, Arthur, Kriketos, Adamandia, and Proietto, Joseph. "Long-Term Persistence of Hormonal Adaptations to Weight Loss." *New England Journal of Medicine* 365 (2011): 1597–1604.

Taylor, Valerie H., McIntyre, Roger S., Remington, Gary, Levitan, Robert D., Stonehocker, Brian, and Sharma, Arya M. "Beyond Pharmacotherapy: Understanding the Links between Obesity and Chronic Mental Illness." *Canadian Journal of Psychiatry* 57, no. 1 (2012): 5–12.

Teitelbaum, Jacob. "Can Childhood Abuse Be Making You Fat?" *Allthingshealing.com.* February 9, 2012. http://www.doctoroz.com/blog/jacob-teitelbaum-md/can-childhood-abuse-be-making-you-fat.

INDEX

About the Author

MARCIA SIROTA, MD, is a board-certified psychiatrist, living in Toronto, Canada. She attended medical school at Memorial University in Newfoundland, Canada, and completed her psychiatry residency in 2000 at Maimonides Medical Center in Brooklyn, New York. She practices individual and group psychotherapy and is a regular contributor to *Moods Magazine* and *The Huffington Post.* She's the founder of the Ruthless Compassion Institute, whose mandate is to promote a philosophy of personal responsibility and empowerment in relationships. Dr. Sirota leads regular workshops for women on overcoming compulsive eating and unblocking creativity. In her spare time, she enjoys salsa dancing.

You can find her online at marciasirotamd.com, @rcinstitute on Twitter, Ruthless Compassion Institute on Facebook, and the ruthlesscompassion channel on YouTube.

About the Series Editor

JULIE SILVER, MD, is Assistant Professor, Harvard Medical School, Department of Physical Medicine and Rehabilitation, and is on the medical staff at Brigham & Women's, Massachusetts General and Spaulding Rehabilitation Hospitals in Boston, Massachusetts. Dr. Silver has authored, edited or co-edited dozens of book, including medical textbooks and consumer health guides. She is also the Chief Editor of Books at Harvard Health Publications. Dr. Silver has won many awards including the American Medical Writers Association Solimene Award for Excellence in Medical Writing and the prestigious Lane Adams Quality of Life Award from the American Cancer Society. Silver is active teaching health care providers how to write and publish, and she is the Director of an annual course offered by the Harvard Medical School Department of Continuing Education titled "Publishing Books, Memoirs and Other Creative Non-Fiction." For more about her work, visit www.JulieSilverMD.com.